The Ultimate Anti-Inflammatory Guide

A Recipe Book to Prepare your Meals in Minutes

Thomas Jollif

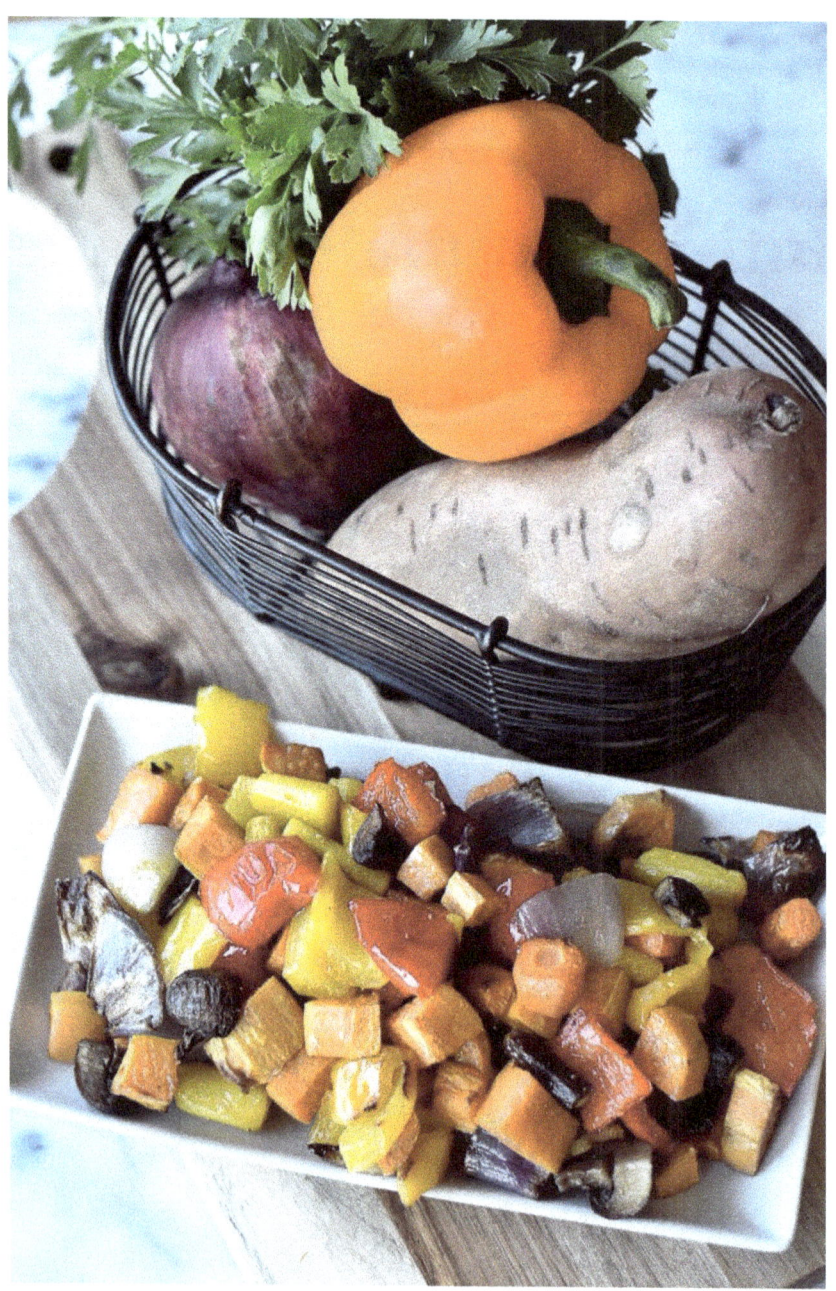

© copyright 2021 – all rights reserved.

the content contained within this book may not be reproduced, duplicated or transmitted without direct written permission from the author or the publisher.

under no circumstances will any blame or legal responsibility be held against the publisher, or author, for any damages, reparation, or monetary loss due to the information contained within this book. either directly or indirectly.

legal notice:

this book is copyright protected. this book is only for personal use. you cannot amend, distribute, sell, use, quote or paraphrase any part, or the content within this book, without the consent of the author or publisher.

disclaimer notice:

please note the information contained within this document is for educational and entertainment purposes only. all effort has been executed to present accurate, up to date, and reliable, complete information. no warranties of any kind are declared or implied. readers acknowledge that the author is not engaging in the rendering of legal, financial, medical or professional advice. the content within this book has been derived from various sources. please consult a licensed professional before attempting any techniques outlined in this book.

by reading this document, the reader agrees that under no circumstances is the author responsible for any losses, direct or indirect, which are incurred as a result of the use of information contained within this document, including, but not limited to, — errors, omissions, or inaccuracies.

Table of Contents

BREAKFASTS 7

Quinoa & Veggie Croquettes 7
Quinoa and Cauliflower Congee 9
Quinoa Breakfast Bowl 12
Raisin Bran Muffins 14
Salmon Burgers 16
Sautéed Veggies on Hot Bagels 18
Savory Bread 20
Savory Veggie Muffins 22
Shirataki Pasta with Avocado and Cream 25
Spicy Ginger Crepes 27
Spicy Marble Eggs 29

SMOOTHIES AND DRINKS 31

Purple Fruit Smoothie 31
Raspberry Banana Smoothie 33
Raspberry Smoothie 35
Spicy Tomato Smoothie 37
Strawberry Oatmeal Smoothie 38
Sweet & Savoury Smoothie 39
Sweet Cranberry Juice 41

SIDES 43

Roasted Portobellos With Rosemary 43
Shoepeg Corn Salad 45
Spiced Sweet Potato Bread 46

Spicy Barley 49

SAUCES AND DRESSINGS 51

Honey Bean Dip 51

Soy with Honey and Ginger Glaze 53

SNACKS 54

Olive and Tomato Balls 54

Oven Crisp Sweet Potato 57

Paleo Ginger Spiced Mixed Nuts 59

Party-Time Chicken Nuggets 61

Peanut Butter and Honey Oat Bars 63

Protein-Packed Croquettes 65

Roasted Beets 67

SOUPS AND STEWS 69

Quick Miso Soup with Wilted 69

Greens 69

Red Lentil Dal 71

Ribollita 73

Rich Onion And Beef Stew 76

Roasted Butternut Squash Apple Soup 78

Russian Cabbage Soup (Shchi) 80

Saffron and Salmon Soup 83

Slow Cooker Lamb & Cauliflower Soup 85

Spicy Asian-Style Soup 87

DESSERTS 89

Pumpkin Ice Cream 89

Pure Avocado Pudding *91*
Raspberry Diluted Frozen Sorbet *93*
Raspberry Gummies *95*
Raspberry Gummies *96*
Raw Black Forest Brownies *98*
Refreshing Raspberry Jelly *100*
Roasted Bananas *102*
Rum Butter Cookies *104*
Sherbet Pineapple *106*

BREAKFASTS

Quinoa & Veggie Croquettes

Time To Prepare: fifteen minutes
Time to Cook: 9 minutes
Yield: Servings 12-fifteen
Ingredients:

- ¼ cup fresh cilantro leaves, chopped
- ¼ teaspoon ground turmeric
- ½ cup frozen peas, thawed
- 1 cup cooked quinoa
- 1 tbsp. essential olive oil
- 1 teaspoon garam masala
- 2 big boiled potatoes, peeled and mashed
- 2 minced garlic cloves
- 2 teaspoons ground cumin
- Freshly ground black pepper, to taste
- Olive oil, for frying
- Salt, to taste

Directions:

1. In a frying pan, warm oil on moderate heat.

2. Put in peas and garlic and sauté for approximately one minute.
3. Move the pea mixture into a big container.
4. Put in the remainder ingredients and mix till well blended.
5. Make equal sized oblong shaped patties from your mixture.
6. In a huge frying pan, heat oil on moderate to high heat.
7. Put in croquettes and fry for approximately 4 minutes per side.

Nutritional Info: Calories: 367 ‖ Fat: 6g ‖ Carbohydrates: 17g ‖ Fiber: 5g ‖ Protein: 22g

Quinoa and Cauliflower Congee

Time To Prepare: ten minutes
Time to Cook: 1 hour
Yield: Servings 8

Ingredients:

- ¼ cup loosely packed cilantro leaves, torn
- ¼ cup loosely packed spearmint leaves, torn
- ¼ cup packed basil leaves, torn
- 1 cauliflower head, minced
- 1 lime, cut into wedges
- 1 tablespoon fish sauce
- 1 tablespoon fresh ginger, grated
- 1 tablespoon olive oil
- 2 garlic cloves, grated
- 2 leeks, minced
- 2 onions, minced
- 2 red chili, minced
- 2 tablespoons brown rice
- 2 tablespoons red quinoa
- 4 eggs, soft-boiled
- 6 cups of water
- For Garnish

- Pinch of white pepper

Directions:

1. Put olive oil into a huge frying pan on moderate heat. Sauté shallots, garlic, and ginger until limp and aromatic; pour into a slow cooker set at moderate heat.
2. Except for decorationes, pour rest of the ingredients into slow cooker; stir. Place the lid on. Cook for around six hours. Turn off heat. Taste; tweak seasoning if required.
3. Ladle congee into separate bowls. Decorate using basil leaves, cilantro leaves, red chilli, and spearmint leaves. Put in 1 piece of soft-boiled egg on top of each; serve with a wedge of lime on the side. Slice egg just before eating so yolk runs into congee. Squeeze lime juice into congee just before eating.

Nutritional Info: Calories: 138 kcal ‖ Protein: 7.23 g ‖ Fat: 7.65 g ‖ Carbohydrates: 10.76 g

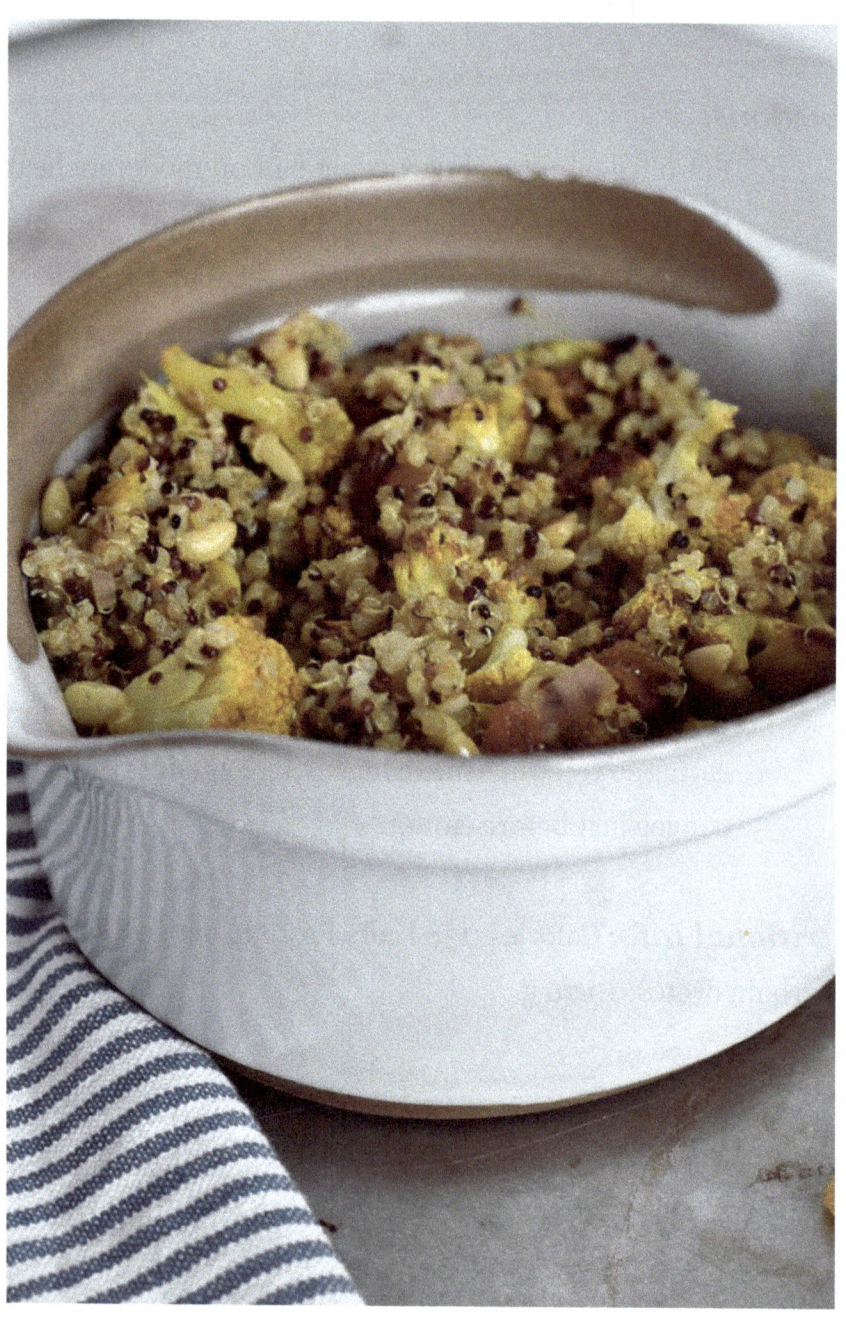

Quinoa Breakfast Bowl

Time To Prepare: thirty minutes
Time to Cook: 0 minutes
Yield: Servings 6

Ingredients:

- ¼ cup Greek yogurt, plain
- ½ tsp. Salt
- 1 cup Baby spinach, chopped
- 1 cup Feta cheese
- 1 Pint Cherry tomatoes, cut in halves
- 1 tsp. Black pepper
- 1 tsp. Garlic, minced
- 1 tsp. Olive oil
- 12 Eggs
- 2 cups Quinoa, cooked

Directions:

1. Mix together the eggs, salt, pepper, garlic, onion powder, and yogurt.
2. Cook the spinach and tomatoes for 5 minutes in the olive oil on moderate heat. Pour in the egg mix and stir until eggs have set to your preferred doneness.

3. Stir in quinoa and feta until they are hot. This will store in your refrigerator for two to three days.

Nutritional Info: Calories 340 ‖ 7.3 grams Fat ‖ 59.4 grams carbs ‖ 6.2 grams fiber ‖ 21.4 grams sugar ‖ 10.5 grams protein.

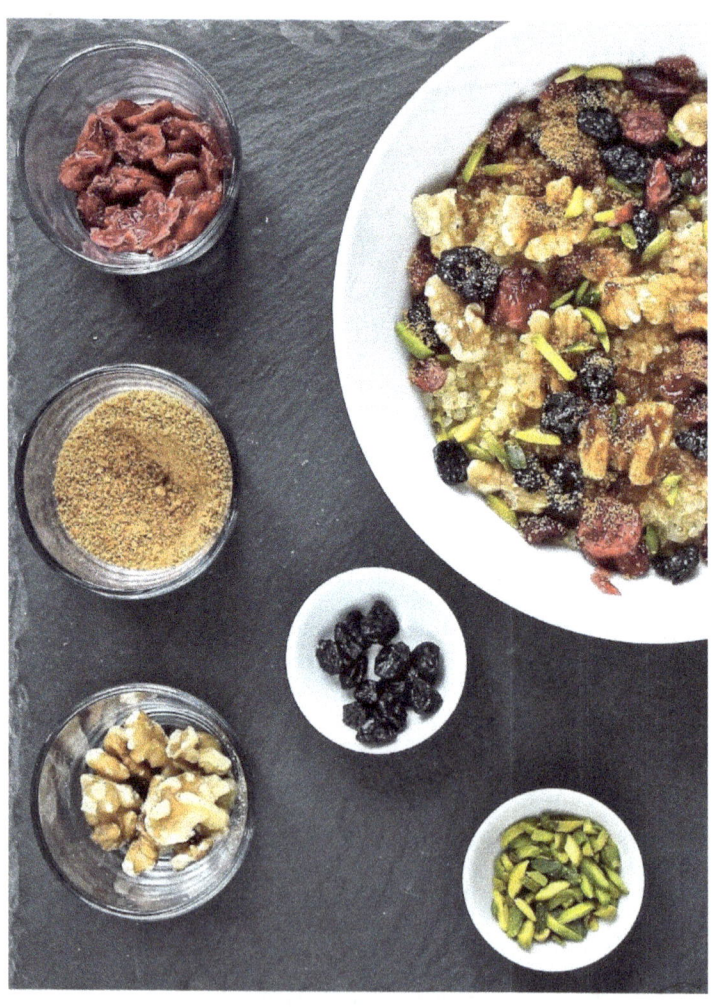

Raisin Bran Muffins

Time To Prepare: fifteen minutes
Time to Cook: thirty minutes
Yield: Servings 36

Ingredients:
- ½ cup vegetable oil
- 1 cup boiling water
- 1 cup bran flakes
- 1 cup sugar
- 1 teaspoon salt
- 1½ cups raisins
- 2 cups buttermilk
- 2 eggs, beaten
- 2½ cups All-Bran cereal
- 2½ cups all-purpose flour
- 2½ teaspoons baking soda

Directions:
1. Set the to 400°F.
2. Grease a muffin tin. Place the boiling water over 1 cup All-Bran, and allow it to sit for about ten minutes.

3. Put the baking soda, flour, and salt in a mixing container then mix, set aside.
4. Mix the oil into the bran and water mixture, then put the rest of the bran, sugar, eggs, and buttermilk.
5. Place the flour mixture to the bran mixture and mix to blend. Mix in the raisins and bran flakes then fill the muffin cups ¾ full with the batter.
6. Bake muffins for about twenty minutes.

Nutritional Info: Calories: 104 ∥ Fat: 4 g ∥ Protein: 2.5 g ∥ Sodium: 187 mg ∥ Fiber: 2 g ∥ Carbohydrates: 17 g

Salmon Burgers

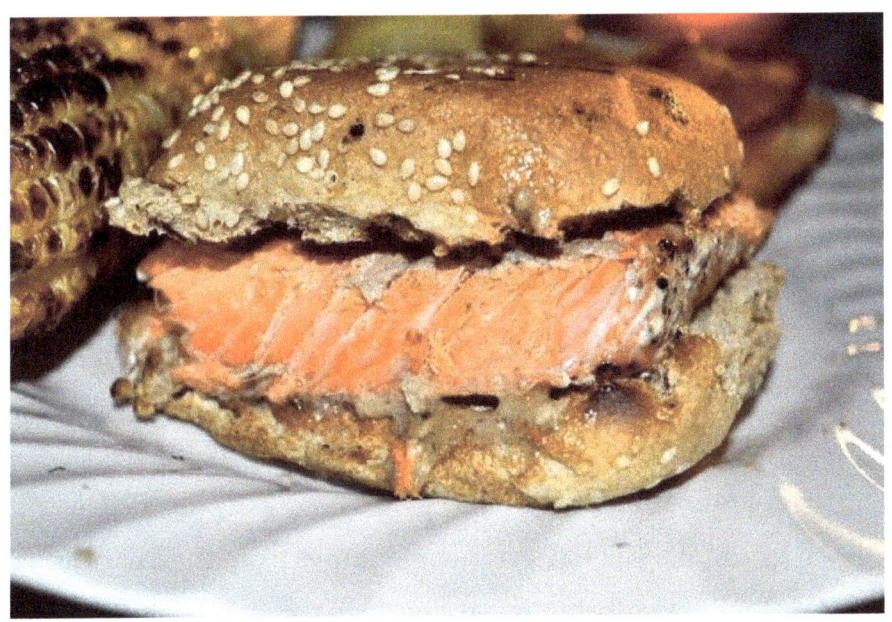

Time To Prepare: fifteen minutes
Time to Cook: 8 minutes
Yield: Servings 3

Ingredients:
- ½ of a medium onion, chopped
- 1 (6-oz. can) skinless, boneless salmon, drained
- 1 celery rib, chopped
- 1 tablespoon dried dill, crushed

- 1 tablespoon plus 1 teaspoon coconut flour
- 1 teaspoon lemon
- 2 big eggs
- 3 tablespoons coconut oil
- Freshly ground black pepper, to taste
- Salt, to taste

Directions:

1. In a substantial container, put in salmon and which has a fork, break it into little pieces.
2. Put in rest of the ingredients excluding the for oil and mix till well blended.
3. Make 6 equal sized small patties from the mixture.
4. In a substantial frying pan, melt coconut oil on moderate to high heat.
5. Cook the patties for about four minutes per side.

Nutritional Info: Calories: 393 ‖ Fat: 12g ‖ Carbohydrates: 19g ‖ Fiber: 5g ‖ Protein: 24g

Sautéed Veggies on Hot Bagels

Time To Prepare: ten minutes
Time to Cook: 16 minutes
Yield: Servings 2

Ingredients:

- ½ onion, cut thin
- 1 clove of garlic, chopped
- 1 tbsp. olive oil
- 1 yellow squash, diced
- 1 zucchini, cut thin
- 2 pcs. tomatoes, cut
- 2 pcs. vegan bagels
- salt and pepper to taste
- vegan butter for spread

Directions:

1. Heat the olive oil on the medium temperature in a cast-iron frying pan.
2. Reduce the heat to moderate-low and sauté the onions for about ten minutes or until the onions start to brown.

3. Turn the heat again to moderate and then put in the diced squash and zucchini to the pan and cook for five minutes. Put in the clove of garlic and cook for one more minute.
4. Throw in the tomato slices to the pan and cook for a minute. Flavor it with pepper and salt and remove the heat.
5. Toast the bagels and cut in half.
6. Spread the bagels lightly with butter and serve with the sautéed veggies on top.

Nutritional Info: Calories: 375 kcal ‖ Protein: 14.69 g ‖ Fat: 11.46 g ‖ Carbohydrates: 54.61 g

Savory Bread

Time To Prepare: ten minutes
Time to Cook: 20 minutes
Yield: Servings 8-10

Ingredients:

- ½ cup plus 1tablespoon almond flour
- 1 cup raw cashew butter
- 1 tablespoon apple cider vinegar
- 1 tablespoon water
- 1 teaspoon ground turmeric
- 1 tsp. baking soda
- 2 big organic eggs
- 2 organic egg whites
- Salt, to taste

Directions:

1. Set the oven to 350F. Grease a loaf pan.
2. In a big pan, combine flour, baking soda, turmeric, and salt.
3. In another container, put in eggs, egg whites, and cashew butter and beat till smooth.
4. Slowly, put in water and beat till well blended.

5. Put in flour mixture and mix till well blended.
6. Mix in apple cider vinegar treatment.
7. Put a combination into prepared loaf pan uniformly.
8. Bake for around 20 minutes or till a toothpick inserted within the middle is released clean.

Nutritional Info: Calories: 347 ‖ Fat: 11g ‖ Carbohydrates: 29g ‖ Fiber: 6g ‖ Protein: 21g

Savory Veggie Muffins

Time To Prepare: fifteen minutes
Time to Cook: 18-23 minutes
Yield: Servings 5

Ingredients:

- ¼ cup concentrate powder
- ½ cup fresh parsley, chopped
- ½ tsp baking soda
- ¾ cup almond meal
- 1 bunch scallion, chopped
- 1 cup coconut butter, softened
- 1½ tablespoons nutritional yeast
- 2 medium carrots, peeled and grated
- 2 tablespoons coconut oil, melted
- 2 teaspoons apple cider vinegar
- 2 teaspoons fresh dill, chopped
- 3 tablespoons fresh lemon juice
- 4 big organic eggs
- Salt, to taste

Directions:

1. Set the oven to 350F. Grease 10 cups of your big muffin tin.

2. In a big container, combine flour, baking soda ‖ Protein: powder, and salt.
3. In another container, put in eggs, nutritional yeast, vinegar, lemon juice, and oil and beat till well blended.
4. Put in coconut butter and beat till the mixture becomes smooth.
5. Put egg mixture into the flour mixture and mix till well blended.
6. Fold in scallion, carts, and parsley.
7. Put the amalgamation into prepared muffin cups uniformly.
8. Bake for approximately 18-23 minutes or till a toothpick inserted inside center comes out clean.

Nutritional Info: Calories: 378 ‖ Fat: 13g ‖ Carbohydrates: 32g ‖ Fiber: 11g ‖ Protein: 32g

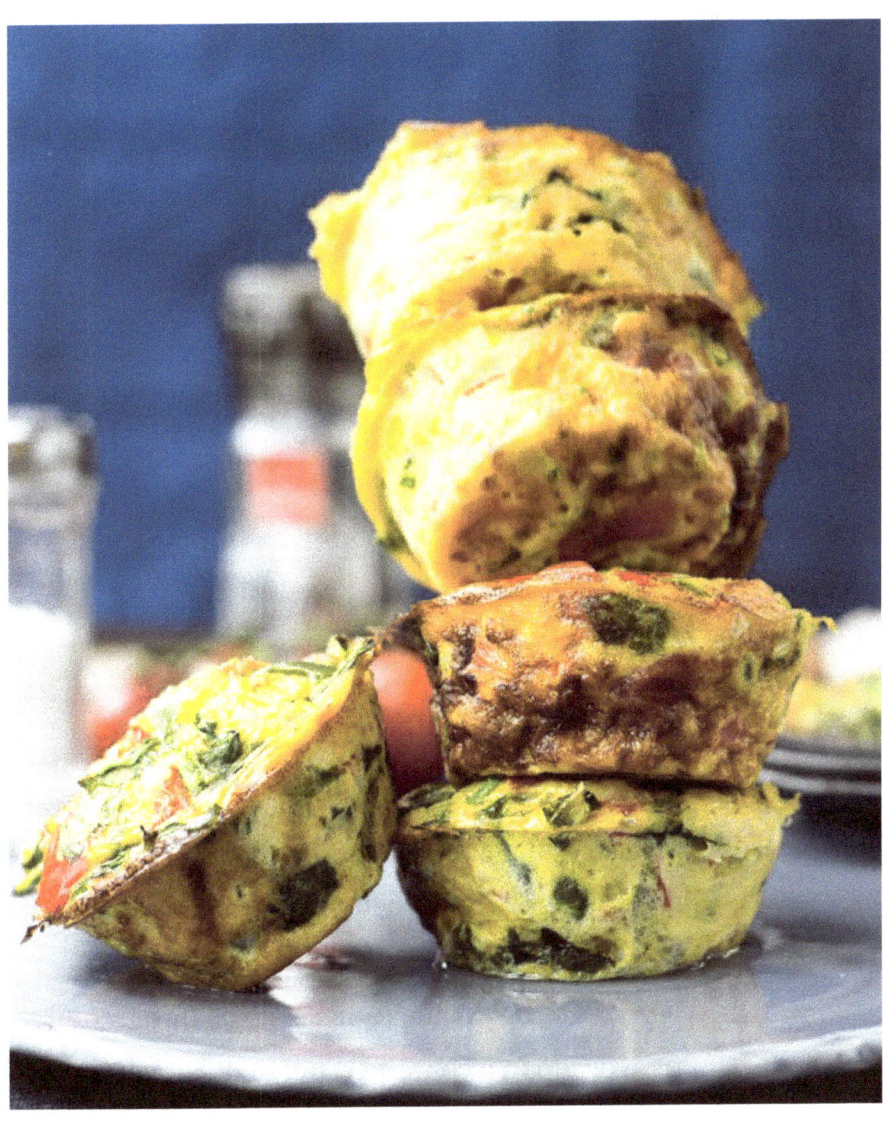

Shirataki Pasta with Avocado and Cream

Time To Prepare: ten minutes
Time to Cook: six minutes
Yield: Servings 2

Ingredients:

- ½ of an avocado
- ½ packet of shirataki noodles, cooked
- ½ tsp cracked black pepper
- ½ tsp dried basil
- ½ tsp salt
- 1/8 cup heavy cream

Directions:

1. Put a medium pot half full with water on moderate heat, bring it to boil, then put in noodles and cook for a couple of minutes.
2. Then drain the noodles and set aside until required.
3. Put avocado in a container, purée it using a fork,
4. Mash avocado in a container, move it to a blender, put in rest of the ingredients, and pulse until the desired smoothness is achieved.

5. Take a frying pan, place it on moderate heat and when hot, put in noodles in it, pour in the avocado mixture, stir thoroughly and cook for a couple of minutes until hot.
6. Serve straight away.

Nutritional Info: Calories 131 ‖ Total Fat: 12.6g ‖ Carbs: 4.9g ‖ Protein: 1.2g ‖ Sugar: 0.3g ‖ Sodium: 588mg

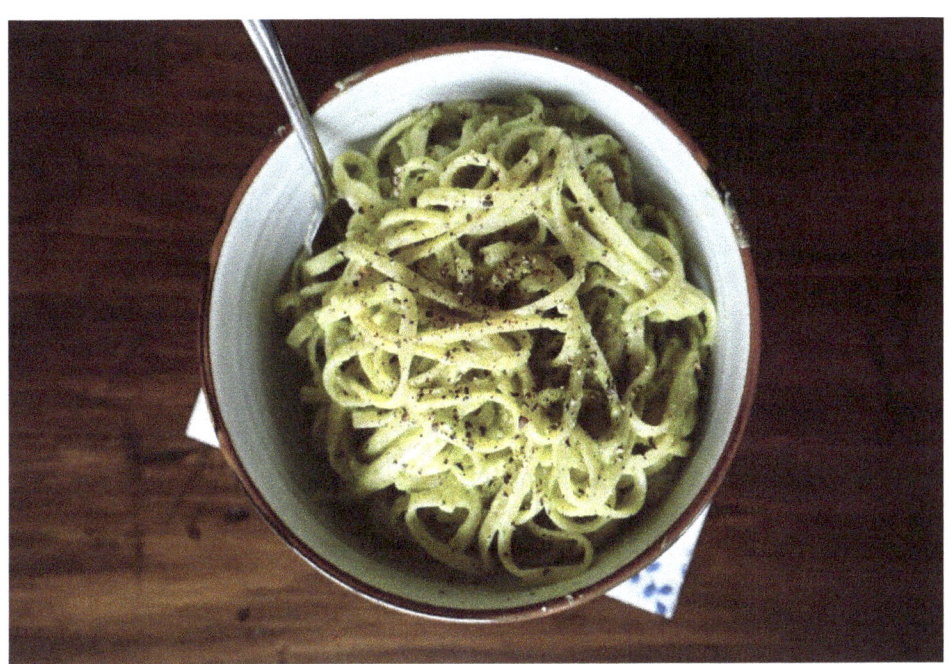

Spicy Ginger Crepes

Time To Prepare: fifteen minutes
Time to Cook: 20 Minutes
Yield: Servings 8

Ingredients:

- ½ teaspoon red chili powder
- 1 (1-inch) fresh ginger piece, grated finely
- 1 1/3 cups chickpea flour
- 1 cup fresh cilantro leaves, chopped
- 1 cup water
- 1 green chili, seeded and chopped finely
- Cooking spray, as required
- Salt, to taste

Directions:

1. In a sizable container, combine flour, chili powder, and salt.
2. Put in ginger, cilantro, and chili and mix thoroughly.
3. Put in water and mix till a uniform mixture form.
4. Keep aside, covered for roughly ½-2 hours.
5. Lightly, grease a substantial nonstick frying pan with cooking spray and heat on moderate to high heat.

6. Put in the desired volume of the mixture and tilt the pan to spread it uniformly inside the frying pan.
7. Cook roughly 10-fifteen seconds per side.
8. Repeat while using the rest of the mixture.

Nutritional Info: Calories: 73 ‖ Fat: 1.3 ‖ Carbohydrates: 11g ‖ Fiber: 2.1g, ‖ Protein: 4.3g

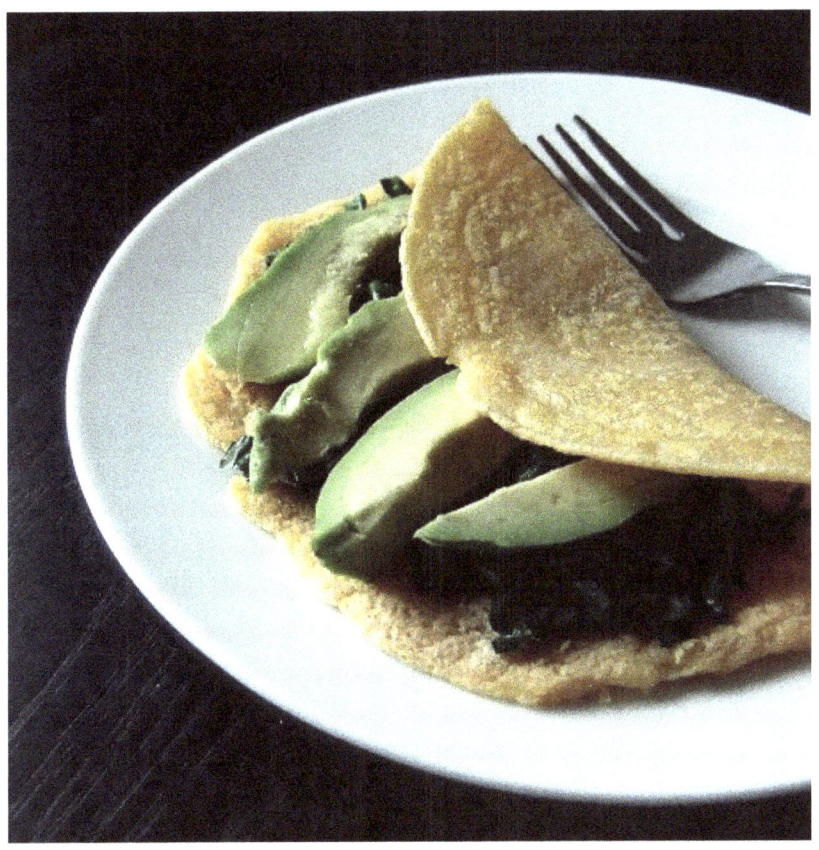

Spicy Marble Eggs

Time To Prepare: fifteen minutes
Time to Cook: 2 hours
Yield: Servings 12

Ingredients:

- 1 dried cinnamon stick, whole
- 1 thumb-sized fresh ginger, unpeeled, crushed
- 1 tsp. dried Szechuan peppercorns
- 1 tsp. salt
- 2 dried bay leaves
- 2 oolong black tea bags
- 3 dried star anise, whole
- 3 Tbsp. brown sugar
- 3 Tbsp. light soy sauce
- 4 cups of water
- 4 Tbsp. dark soy sauce
- 6 medium-boiled eggs, unpeeled, cooled
- For the Marinade

Directions:

1. Use the back of a spoon to crack eggshells in places to create a spider web effect. Do not peel. Set aside until needed.

2. Pour marinade into big Dutch oven set using high heat. Put lid partly on. Bring water to a rolling boil, approximately five minutes. Turn off heat.
3. Close the lid. Steep ingredients for about ten minutes.
4. Use a slotted spoon to fish out and discard solids. Cool marinade completely to room proceeding.
5. Put eggs into an airtight non-reactive container just small enough to tightly fit all these in.
6. Pour in marinade. Eggs must be completely immersed in liquid. Discard leftover marinade, if any. Coat container rim with generous layers of saran wrap. Secure container lid.
7. Chill eggs for one day before you use.
8. Extract eggs and drain each piece well before you use, but keep the rest immersed in the marinade.

Nutritional Info: Calories: 75 kcal ‖ Protein: 4.05 g ‖ Fat: 4.36 g ‖ Carbohydrates: 4.83 g

SMOOTHIES AND DRINKS

Purple Fruit Smoothie

Time To Prepare: ten minutes
Time to Cook: 0 minutes
Yield: Servings 1

Ingredients:
- 2 frozen bananas, cut in chunks
- 1 cup orange juice
- 1 tbsp. honey, optional
- 1 tsp. vanilla extract, optional
- 1/2 cup frozen blueberries

Directions:
1. Put in everything to a blender jug.
2. Cover the jug firmly.
3. Blend until the desired smoothness is achieved. Serve and enjoy!

Nutritional Info: Calories: 133 ‖ Fat: 1.1 g ‖ Protein: 3.6 g ‖ Carbohydrates: 7.6 g ‖ Fiber: 1.3 g

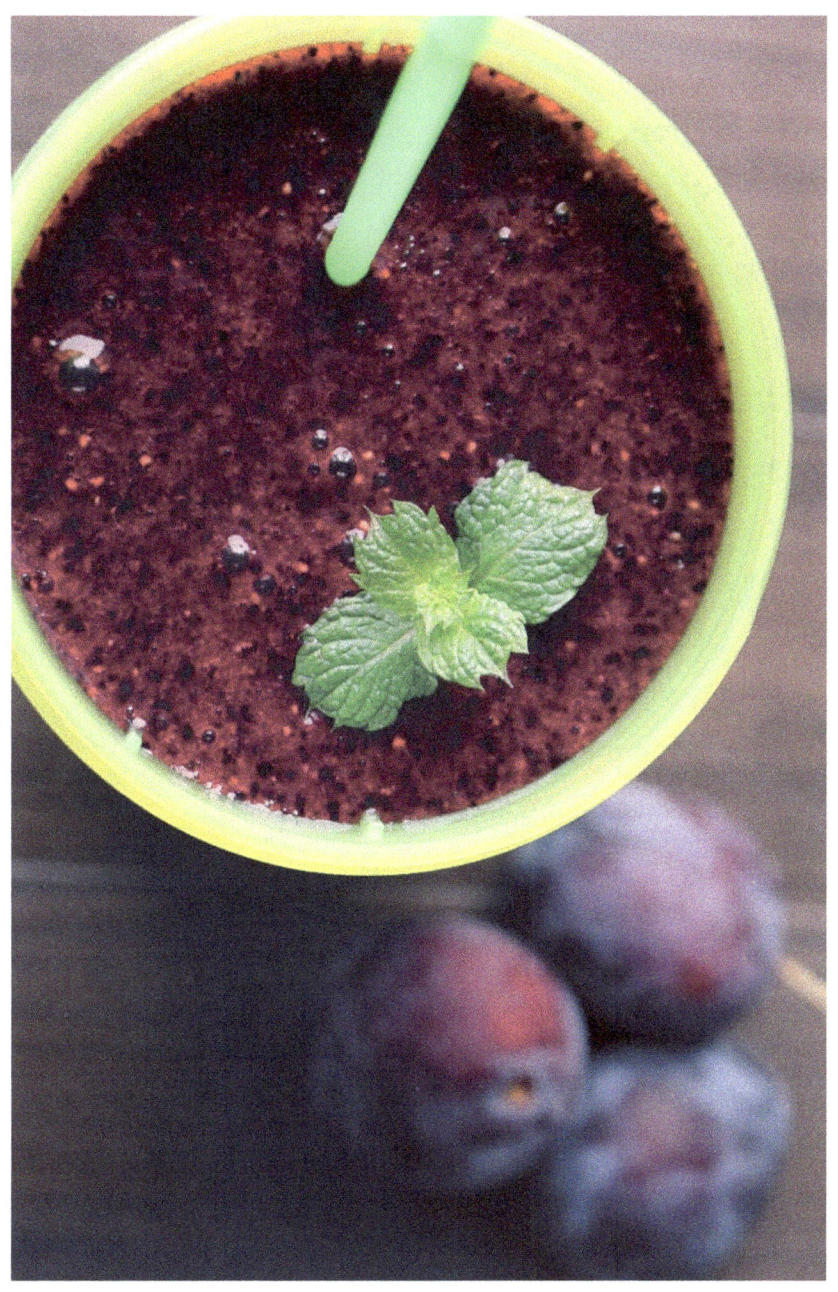

Raspberry Banana Smoothie

Time To Prepare: ten minutes
Time to Cook: 0 minutes
Yield: Servings 1

Ingredients:

- 1 banana
- 1 cup almond milk
- 1 cup frozen raspberries
- 1 cup raspberry yogurt
- 1 tbsp. flaxseed meal
- 1/4 cup Concord grape juice
- 1/4 cup rolled oats
- 16 whole almonds

Directions:

1. Put in everything to a blender jug.
2. Cover the jug firmly.
3. Blend until the desired smoothness is achieved and then serve. Enjoy!

Nutritional Info: Calories: 214 ‖ Fat: 0.4 g ‖ Protein: 5.6 g ‖ Carbohydrates: 8 g ‖ Fiber: 2.3 g

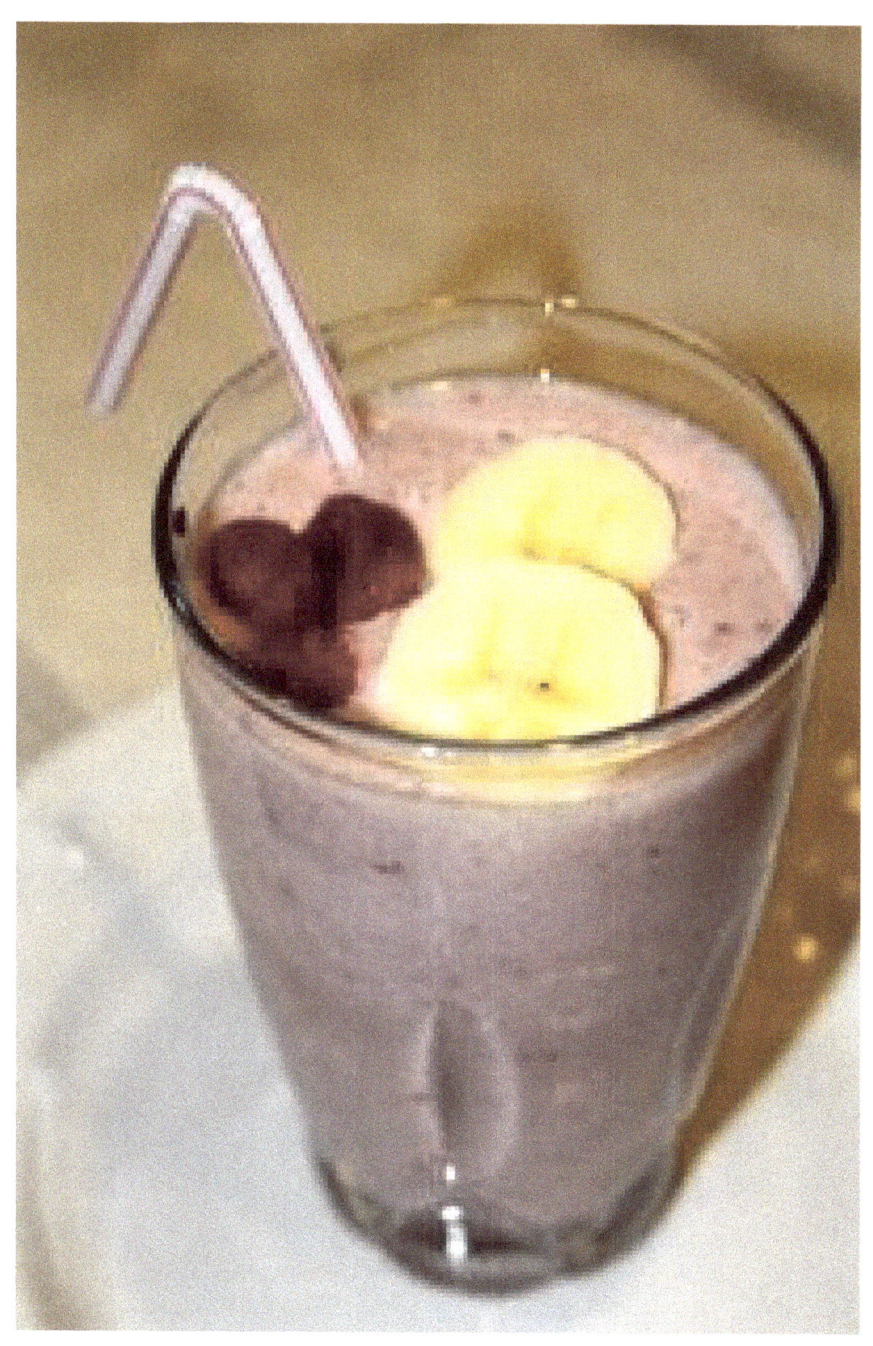

Raspberry Smoothie

Time To Prepare: ten minutes
Time to Cook: 0 minutes
Yield: Servings 2

Ingredients:

- 1 avocado, pitted and peeled
- 1/2 cup raspberries
- 3/4 cup raspberry juice
- 3/4 cup orange juice

Directions:

1. In your blender, combine the avocado with the raspberry juice, orange juice, and raspberries.
2. Pulse thoroughly, split into 2 glasses, before you serve. Enjoy!

Nutritional Info: Calories: 125 ‖ Fat: 11 g ‖ Protein: 3 g ‖ Carbohydrates: 9 g ‖ Fiber: 7 g

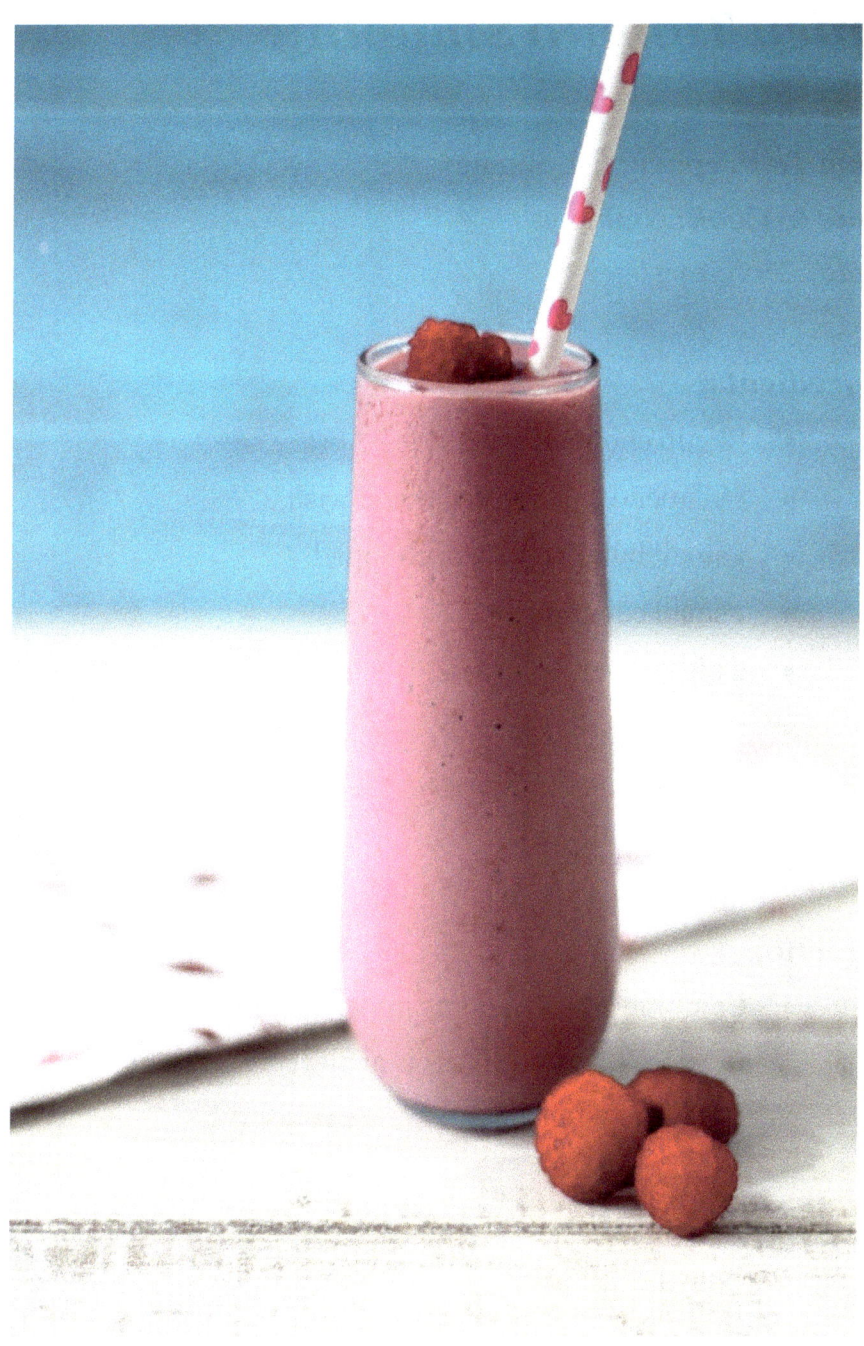

Spicy Tomato Smoothie

Time To Prepare: five minutes
Time to Cook: 0 minutes
Yield: Servings 2

Ingredients:

- ¼ cup chopped red onion
- 1 jalapeño, cut, deseed if you wish
- 1 small bunch cilantro, chopped
- 1 small cucumber
- 2 big carrots, chopped
- 2 cloves garlic, peeled
- 6 small vine tomatoes
- Juice of 2 limes

Directions:

1. Combine all ingredients into a blender and blend until the desired smoothness is achieved.
2. Pour into 2 tall glasses before you serve.

Nutritional Info: Calories: 269 kcal ∥ Protein: 24.87 g ∥ Fat: 8.71 g ∥ Carbohydrates: 26.89 g

Strawberry Oatmeal Smoothie

Time To Prepare: ten minutes
Time to Cook: 0 minutes
Yield: Servings 1

Ingredients:
- 1 cup soy milk
- 1 banana, broken into chunks
- 14 frozen strawberries
- 1/2 cup rolled oats
- 1/2 tsp. vanilla extract
- 1 1/2 tsp. honey

Directions:
1. Put in everything to a blender jug.
2. Cover the jug firmly.
3. Blend until the desired smoothness is achieved. Serve and enjoy!

Nutritional Info: Calories: 172 ‖ Fat: 0.4 g ‖ Protein: 5.6 g ‖ Carbohydrates: 8 g ‖ Fiber: 2 g

Sweet & Savoury Smoothie

Time To Prepare: five minutes
Time to Cook: 0 minutes
Yield: Servings 2

Ingredients:

- 1 apple, peeled and cut
- 1 banana, peeled and cut
- 1 cup of almond or soy milk
- 1 cup of fresh pineapple, peeled and cut
- 1 tbsp. of lemon juice
- 1/2 tbsp. of ginger, grated
- 1/4 tsp of ground turmeric
- 2 cups of carrots, peeled and cut
- 2 cups of filtered water.

Directions:

1. Blend carrots and water to make a pureed carrot juice.
2. Pour into a Mason jar or sealable container, cover, and store in the refrigerator.
3. When done, put in the rest of the smoothie ingredients to a blender or juicer until the desired smoothness is achieved.

4. Put in the carrot juice in at the end, blending meticulously until the desired smoothness is achieved.
5. Serve with or without ice.

Nutritional Info: Calories: 225 kcal ‖ Protein: 6.03 g ‖ Fat: 5.78 g ‖ Carbohydrates: 39.93 g

Sweet Cranberry Juice

Time To Prepare: five minutes
Time to Cook: 8 minutes
Yield: Servings 4

Ingredients:

- ½ cup honey
- 1 cinnamon stick
- 1 gallon filtered water
- 4 cups fresh cranberries
- Juice of 1 lemon

Directions:

1. Put in cranberries, ½ of water, cinnamon cling to the instant pot.
2. Secure the lid. Cook on HIGH pressure 8 minutes.
3. Depressurize naturally.
4. Once cool, strain liquid. Put in remaining water.
5. Mix in honey and lemon. Cool thoroughly.
6. Chill before you serve.

Nutritional Info: Calories: 184 ‖ Fat: 0g ‖ Carbohydrates: 49g ‖ Protein: 1g

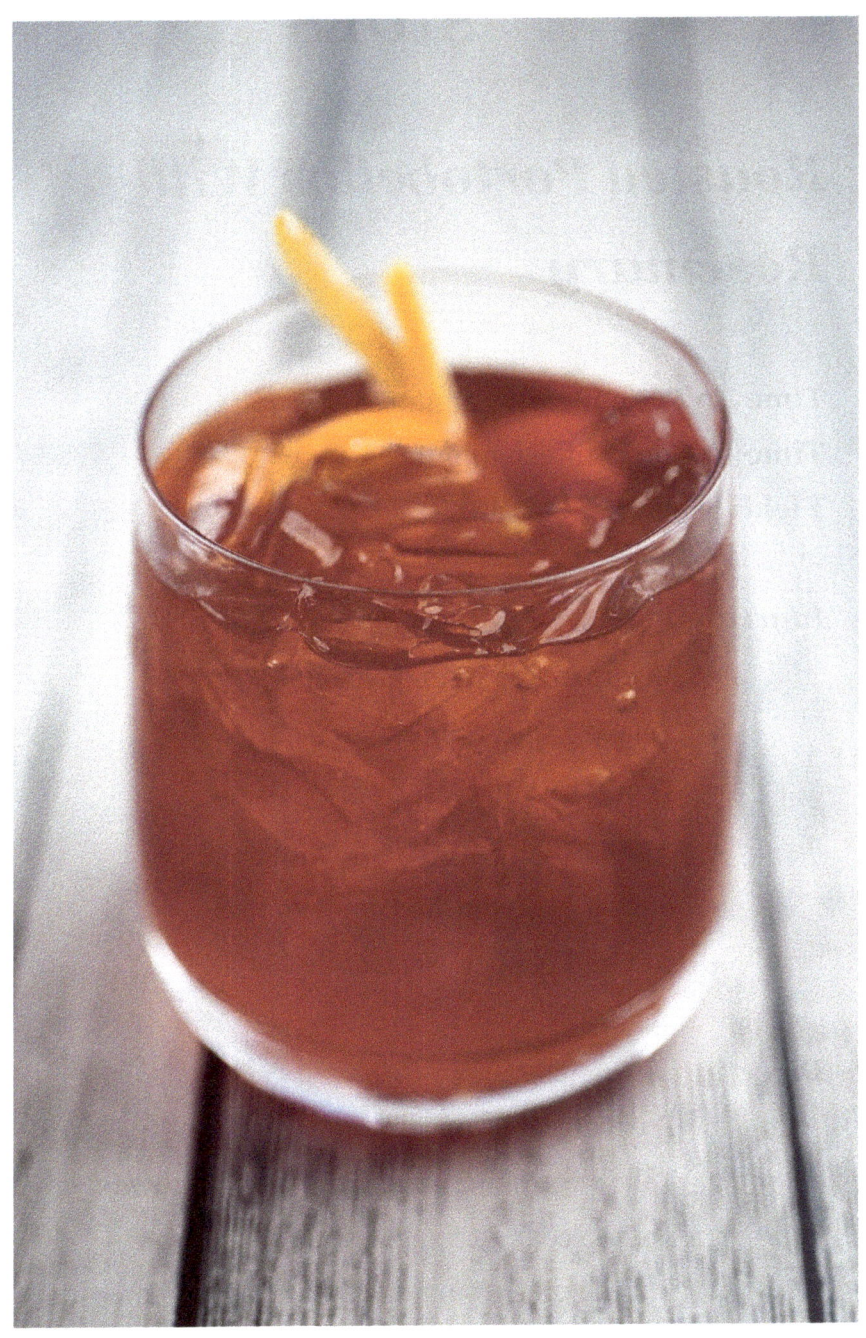

SIDES

Roasted Portobellos With Rosemary

Time To Prepare: five minutes
Time to Cook: fifteen minutes
Yield: Servings 4

Ingredients:

- ¼ cup extra virgin olive oil
- 1 clove garlic, minced
- 1 sprig rosemary, torn
- 2 tablespoons fresh lemon juice
- 8 portobello mushroom, trimmed
- Salt and pepper, to taste

Directions:

1. Preheat the oven to 450 degrees F
2. Take a container and put in all ingredients
3. Toss to coat
4. Put the mushroom in a baking sheet stem side up
5. Roast in your oven for fifteen minutes

6. Serve and enjoy!

Nutritional Info: ‖ Calories: 63 ‖ Fat: 6g ‖ Carbohydrates: 2g ‖ Protein:1g

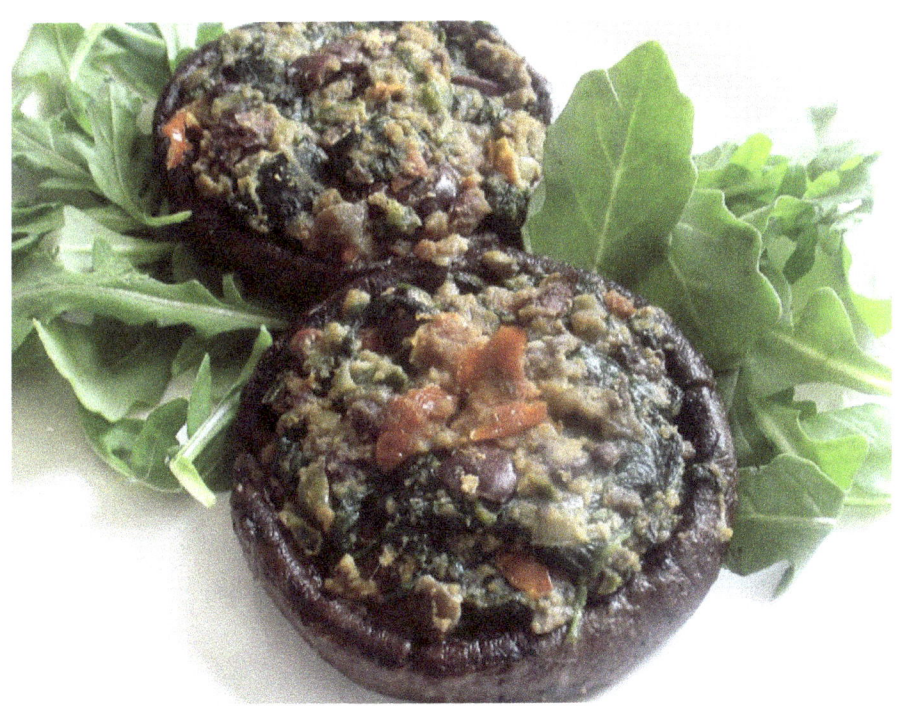

Shoepeg Corn Salad

Time To Prepare: ten minutes
Time to Cook: 0 minute
Yield: Servings 4

Ingredients:

- ¼ cup Greek yogurt
- ½ cup cherry tomatoes halved
- 1 cup shoepeg corn, drained
- 1 jalapeno pepper, chopped
- 1 tablespoon chives, chopped
- 1 tablespoon lemon juice
- 3 tablespoons fresh cilantro, chopped

Directions:

1. In the salad container, mix up together shoepeg corn, cherry tomatoes, jalapeno pepper, chives, and fresh cilantro.
2. Put in lemon juice and Greek yogurt. Mix yo the salad well.
3. Put in your fridge and store it for maximum 1 day.

Nutritional Info: Calories 49 ‖ Fat: 0.7 ‖ Fiber: 1.2 ‖ Carbs: 9.4 ‖ Protein: 2.7

Spiced Sweet Potato Bread

Time To Prepare: fifteen minutes
Time to Cook: 45-55 minutes
Yield: Servings 2

Ingredients:
For dry Ingredients :

- ¼ teaspoon sea salt
- 1 cup coconut flour
- 1 teaspoon ground mace
- 2 tablespoons ground cinnamon
- 2 teaspoons baking powder
- 2 teaspoons baking soda
- 2 teaspoons ground nutmeg

Wet Ingredients:

- 1 cup almond butter
- 2 teaspoons organic almond extract
- 4 big sweet potatoes, peeled, thinly cut
- 4 tablespoons coconut oil
- 8 big eggs
- 8 tablespoons melted grass fed butter, unsalted

Directions:

1. Grease 2 loaf pans of 9 x 5 inches with coconut oil. Coat the bottom of the pan using parchment paper. Set aside.
2. Put a medium deep cooking pan on moderate heat. Put in sweet potatoes. Pour enough water to immerse the sweet potatoes. Cook until the sweet potatoes are soft.
3. Remove the heat and drain the sweet potatoes.
4. Put in the sweet potatoes back into the pan. Mash with a potato masher until the desired smoothness is achieved. Allow it to cool completely.
5. Put all together the dry ingredients into a container and mix thoroughly.
6. Put in eggs into a big container and whisk well. Put in sweet potatoes, butter, almond extract and almond butter and whisk until well blended.
7. Put in the dry ingredients into the container of wet ingredients and whisk until well blended.
8. Split the batter into the prepared loaf pans.
9. Bake in a preheated oven at 350°F for approximately 45 -55 minutes or a toothpick when inserted in the middle of the loaf comes out clean.
10. Remove from oven and cool to room temperature.
11. Slice using a sharp knife into slices of 1-inch thickness.

Nutritional Info: ‖ Calories: 1738 kcal ‖ Protein: 27 g ‖ Fat: 145.92 g ‖ Carbohydrates: 89.58 g

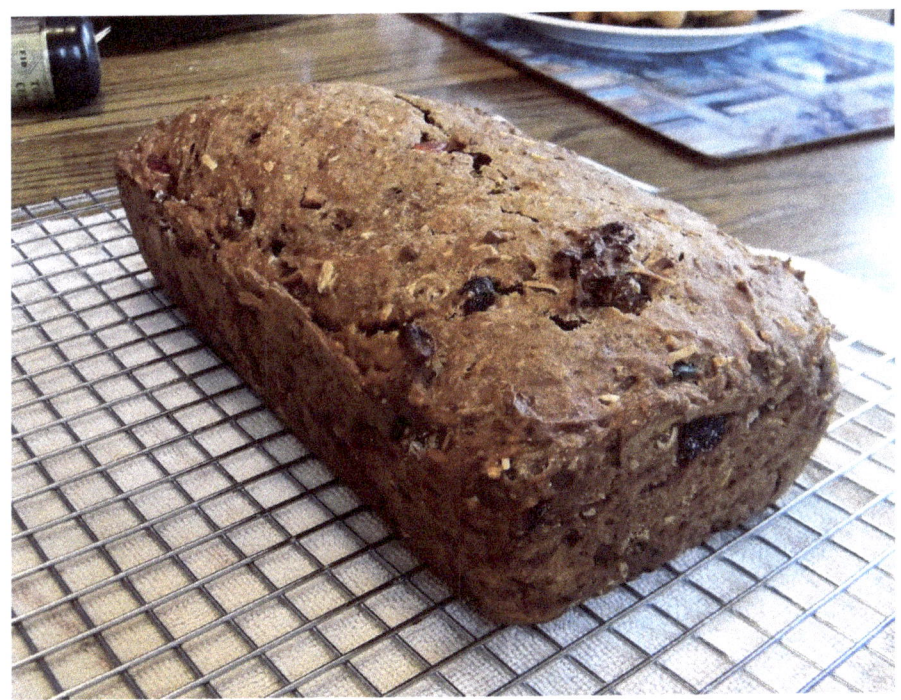

Spicy Barley

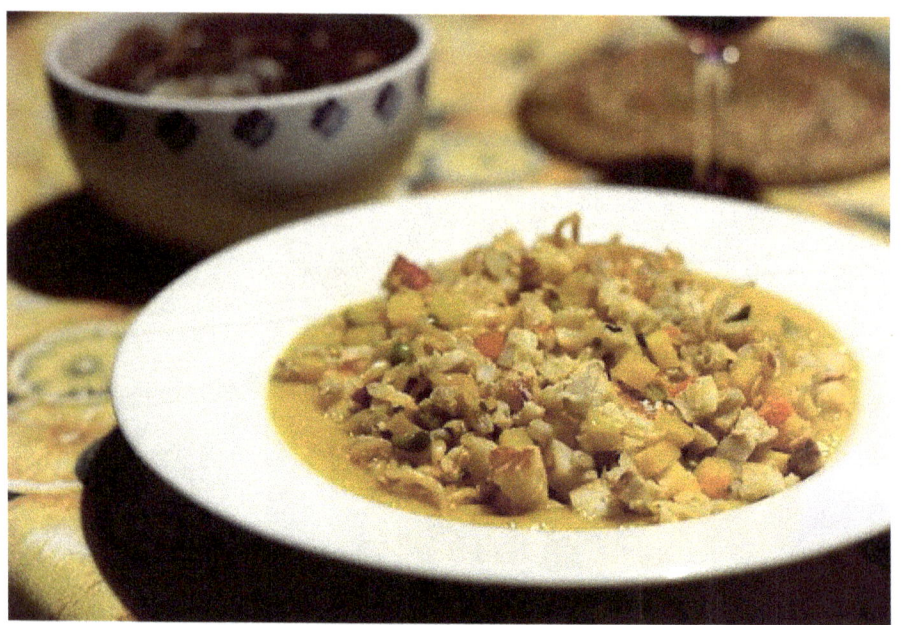

Time To Prepare: seven minutes
Time to Cook: 42 minutes
Yield: Servings 5

Ingredients:

- ½ teaspoon cayenne pepper
- ½ teaspoon chili pepper
- ½ teaspoon ground black pepper
- 1 cup barley

- 1 teaspoon butter
- 1 teaspoon olive oil
- 1 teaspoon salt
- 3 cups chicken stock

Directions:
1. Put barley and olive oil in the pan.
2. Roast barley on high heat for a minute. Stir it well.
3. Then put in salt, chili pepper, ground black pepper, cayenne pepper, and butter.
4. Put in chicken stock.
5. Close the lid and cook barley for forty minutes over the medium-low heat.

Nutritional Info: Calories 152 ‖ Fat: 2.9 ‖ Fiber: 6.5 ‖ Carbs: 27.8 ‖ Protein: 5.1

SAUCES AND DRESSINGS

Honey Bean Dip

Time To Prepare: five minutes
Time to Cook: 0 minutes
Yield: Servings 3-4
Ingredients:

- ¼ teaspoon ground cumin
- ¼ teaspoon salt
- 1 (14-ounce) can each of kidney beans and black beans
- 1 tablespoon apple cider vinegar
- 1 teaspoon lime juice
- 2 cherry tomatoes
- 2 garlic cloves
- 2 tablespoons filtered water
- 2 teaspoons raw honey
- Freshly ground black pepper to taste
- Pinch cayenne pepper to taste

Directions:

1. In a blender or food processor, put together the beans, garlic, tomatoes, water, vinegar, honey, lime juice, cumin, salt, cayenne pepper, and black pepper.

2. Blend until it becomes smooth. Put in the mix in a container.
3. Cover and place in your fridge to chill. You can place in your fridge for maximum 5 days.

Nutritional Info: Calories 158 ‖ Fat: 1g ‖ Carbohydrates: 33g ‖ Fiber: 8g ‖ Protein: 9g

Soy with Honey and Ginger Glaze

Time To Prepare: ten minutes
Time to Cook: 0 minutes
Yield: Servings 2-4

Ingredients:

- ¼ cup of honey
- 1 tbsp. of rice vinegar
- 1 tsp of freshly grated ginger
- 2 tbsp. gluten-free soy sauce

Directions:

1. Put all together the ingredients into a small container and whisk well.
2. Serve with a vegetables, chickens, or seafood.
3. Keep the glaze in a mason jar, firmly covered, and place in your fridge for maximum four days.

Nutritional Info: ‖ Calories: 90 kcal ‖ Protein: 2.32 g ‖ Fat: 1.54 g ‖ Carbohydrates: 17.99 g

SNACKS

Olive and Tomato Balls

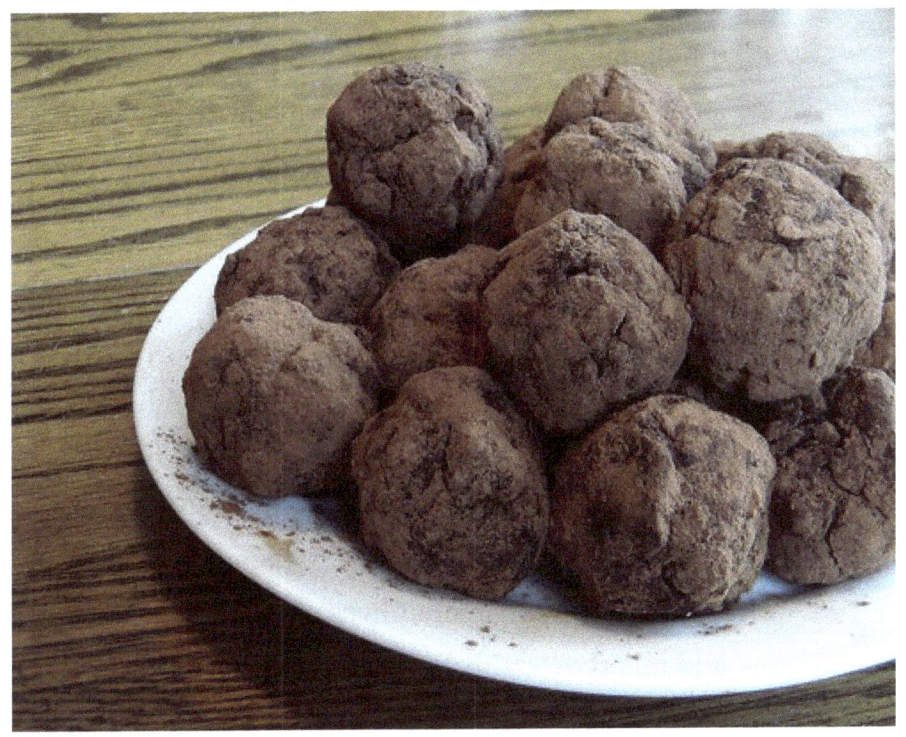

Time To Prepare: ten minutes
Time to Cook: thirty-five minutes
Yield: Servings 5
Ingredients:
- .25 cup Coconut oil

- .25 tsp. Salt
- .5 cup Cream cheese
- 2 cloves Garlic, crushed
- 2 tbsp. Basil, chopped
- 2 tbsp. Oregano, chopped
- 2 tbsp. Thyme, chopped
- 4 Kalamata olives, pitted
- 4 pcs. Sun-dried tomatoes, drained
- 5 tbsp. Parmesan cheese, grated
- Black pepper (as you wish)

Directions:

1. Cut the coconut oil, put in it to a small mixing container with the cream cheese, and allow them to tenderize for approximately 30 minutes. Mash together and mix thoroughly to blend.
2. Put in in the Kalamata olives and sun-dried tomatoes and mix thoroughly before you put in in the herbs and seasonings. Mix meticulously before placing the mixing container in your fridge to allow the results to solidify.
3. Once it has solidified, make the mixture into a total of 5 balls using an ice cream scoop. Roll each of the finished balls into the parmesan cheese before plating.

4. Stored the extra's in your refrigerator in an air-tight container for maximum 7 days.

Nutritional Info: ‖ Calories: 212 kcal ‖ Protein: 4.77 g ‖ Fat: 20.75 g ‖ Carbohydrates: 3.13 g

Oven Crisp Sweet Potato

Time To Prepare: ten minutes
Time to Cook: twenty minutes
Yield: Servings 2

Ingredients:

- 1 moderate-sized sweet potato, raw
- 1 teaspoon coconut oil
- 1 teaspoon sugar

Directions:

1. Preheat your oven to 160C.
2. Using a mandolin slicer or a peeler, slice the sweet potato into thin chips or strips. Rinse and pat dry.
3. Sprinkle the coconut oil over the potatoes. Toss until all chips are coated.
4. Position in an oven baking sheet. Bake for about ten minutes. Check the crispiness. If it is not that crunchy enough, bake for an extra five or 10 minutes or until the chips attain the crispiness desired.
5. Take out the crunchy sweet potatoes. Drizzle with sugar before you serve.

Nutritional Info: ‖ Calories: 123 kcal ‖ Protein: 4.23 g ‖ Fat: 5.39 g ‖ Carbohydrates: 14.63 g

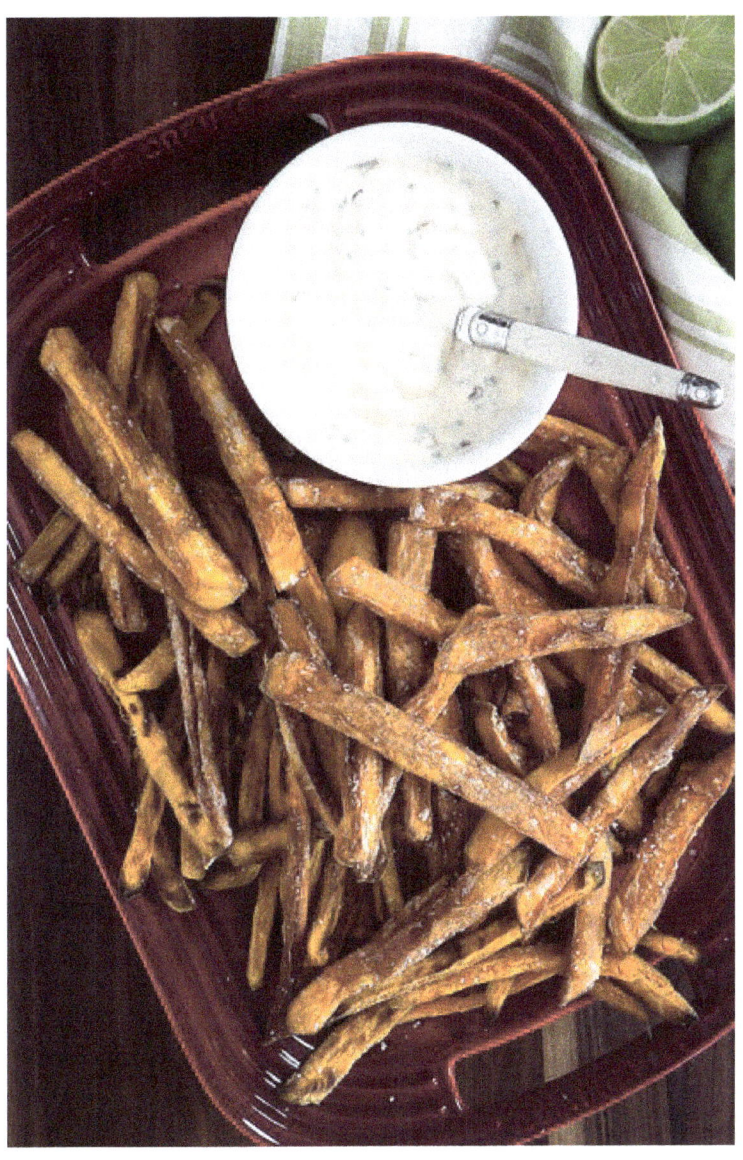

Paleo Ginger Spiced Mixed Nuts

Time To Prepare: five minutes
Time to Cook: forty minutes
Yield: Servings 8

Ingredients:

- ½ tsp. Fine sea salt
- ½ tsp. Vietnamese cinnamon
- 1 tsp. Grated fresh ginger
- 2 cups Mix nuts; Cashew, goji berries, raw almonds, pumpkin seeds, etc.
- 2 Large Egg,
- Coconut oil spray
- Egg whites

Directions:

1. Prepare the oven by preheating to 250°F.
2. Whisk egg whites in a container until it gets fluffy. Pour in sea salt, grated ginger, and Vietnamese cinnamon. Whisk until it's one big mix.
3. Pour in the mixed nuts and stir to combine.
4. Coat the parchment-lined baking sheet with coconut oil spray and spread the nut mixture all across the baking sheet.

5. Allow it to bake for approximately twenty minutes, rotate the sheet then bake for another twenty minutes.
6. Take off the baking sheet from the oven and leave to cool.
7. Once it's fully cool and hard, break them into bits with clean hands.
8. Serve or store.

Nutritional Info: ‖ Calories: 212 kcal ‖ Protein: 6.92 g ‖ Fat: 17.3 g ‖ Carbohydrates: 10.05 g

Party-Time Chicken Nuggets

Time To Prepare: ten minutes
Time to Cook: twenty-five minutes
Yield: Servings 6

Ingredients:

- ½ cup tapioca flour
- ½ tsp. of garlic powder
- ½ tsp. of onion powder
- ½ tsp. of paprika
- 1½ cups of blanched almond flour
- 2 (6-ounce) grass-fed skinless, boneless chicken breasts
- 2 big organic eggs
- Freshly ground black pepper, to taste
- Salt, to taste

Directions:

1. Set the oven to 400F then grease a big baking sheet.
2. With a rolling pin, roll the chicken breasts to a uniform thickness.
3. Cut each breast into bite-sized pieces.
4. In a shallow dish, crack the eggs and beat thoroughly.

5. In another shallow dish, combine flours and spices.
6. Immerse the chicken nuggets in beaten eggs.
7. Then roll in flour mixture completely.
8. Position the nuggets onto the readied baking sheet in a single layer.
9. Bake for approximately 10-twelve minutes, turning once after five minutes.

Nutritional Info: ‖ Calories: 312 ‖ Fat: 17.8g ‖ Carbohydrates: 15.4g ‖ Protein: 23.6g ‖ Fiber: 3.2g

Peanut Butter and Honey Oat Bars

Time To Prepare: ten minutes
Time to Cook: twenty-five minutes
Yield: Servings 18

Ingredients:

- ¼ cup honey
- ¼ cup honey roasted peanuts, chopped
- ¼ teaspoon cinnamon powder
- ¼ teaspoon vanilla extract
- 1 cup oats
- 2 teaspoons coconut oil
- 3 tablespoons peanut butter

Directions:

1. Coat a small baking pan using a parchment paper such that the parchment paper is hanging over the sides of the baking pan.
2. Put in honey, oil, and peanut butter into a microwave-safe container. Microwave on High for around 20 -half a minute or until the peanut butter melts completely.

If it takes longer than half a minute, stir and cook in increments of 10 seconds, stirring every time.
3. Remove from the microwave and put in the remaining ingredients. Mix thoroughly and pour into the readied baking pan. Spread the mixture and press using a spatula.
4. Bake in a preheated oven 300° F for approximately twenty minutes or until the top is light brown.
5. Take out of the oven and press once once more.
6. Cool for a while and slice.
7. Cool thoroughly before you serve.
8. Move leftover bars into an airtight container. Place in your fridge until use.

Nutritional Info: ‖ Calories: 44 kcal ‖ Protein: 1.47 g ‖ Fat: 1.69 g ‖ Carbohydrates: 8.06 g

Protein-Packed Croquettes

Time To Prepare: ten minutes
Time to Cook: five minutes
Yield: Servings 12

Ingredients:
- ¼ cup of chopped fresh cilantro leaves
- ¼ cup plus 1 tbsp. of olive oil, divided
- ¼ tsp. of ground turmeric
- ½ cup of thawed frozen peas
- ½ tsp. of paprika
- 1 cup of cooked quinoa
- 2 big peeled and mashed boiled potatoes
- 2 minced garlic cloves
- 2 tsp. of ground cumin
- Freshly ground black pepper, to taste
- Salt, to taste

Directions:
1. In a frying pan, heat 1 tbsp. of oil on moderate heat.
2. Put in peas and garlic and sauté for approximately one minute.
3. Move the peas mixture into a big container.

4. Put rest of the ingredients then mix till well blended.
5. Make equal sized oblong shaped patties from the mixture.
6. In a huge frying pan, warm remaining oil on moderate to high heat.
7. Put in croquettes in batches and fry for approximately 4 minutes per side.

Nutritional Info: ‖ Calories: 152 ‖ Fat: 6.9g ‖ Carbohydrates: 20.1g ‖ Protein: 3.5g ‖ Fiber: 2.9g

Roasted Beets

Time To Prepare: ten minutes
Time to Cook: 35-45 minutes
Yield: Servings 6

Ingredients:

- 1 tablespoon of coconut oil, melted
- 1 teaspoon of salt
- 2 and a ½ pounds of beets, peeled and diced

Directions:

1. Preheat your oven to 400°F.
2. Spread the beets onto a baking sheet and sprinkle with melted coconut oil.
3. Put in salt and mix thoroughly.
4. Roast the beets in your oven for 35-45 minutes, until the beets are tender.

Nutritional Info: ‖ Total Carbohydrates: 7g ‖ Fiber: 2g ‖ Net Carbohydrates: ‖ Protein: 1g ‖ Total Fat: 4g ‖ Calories: 59

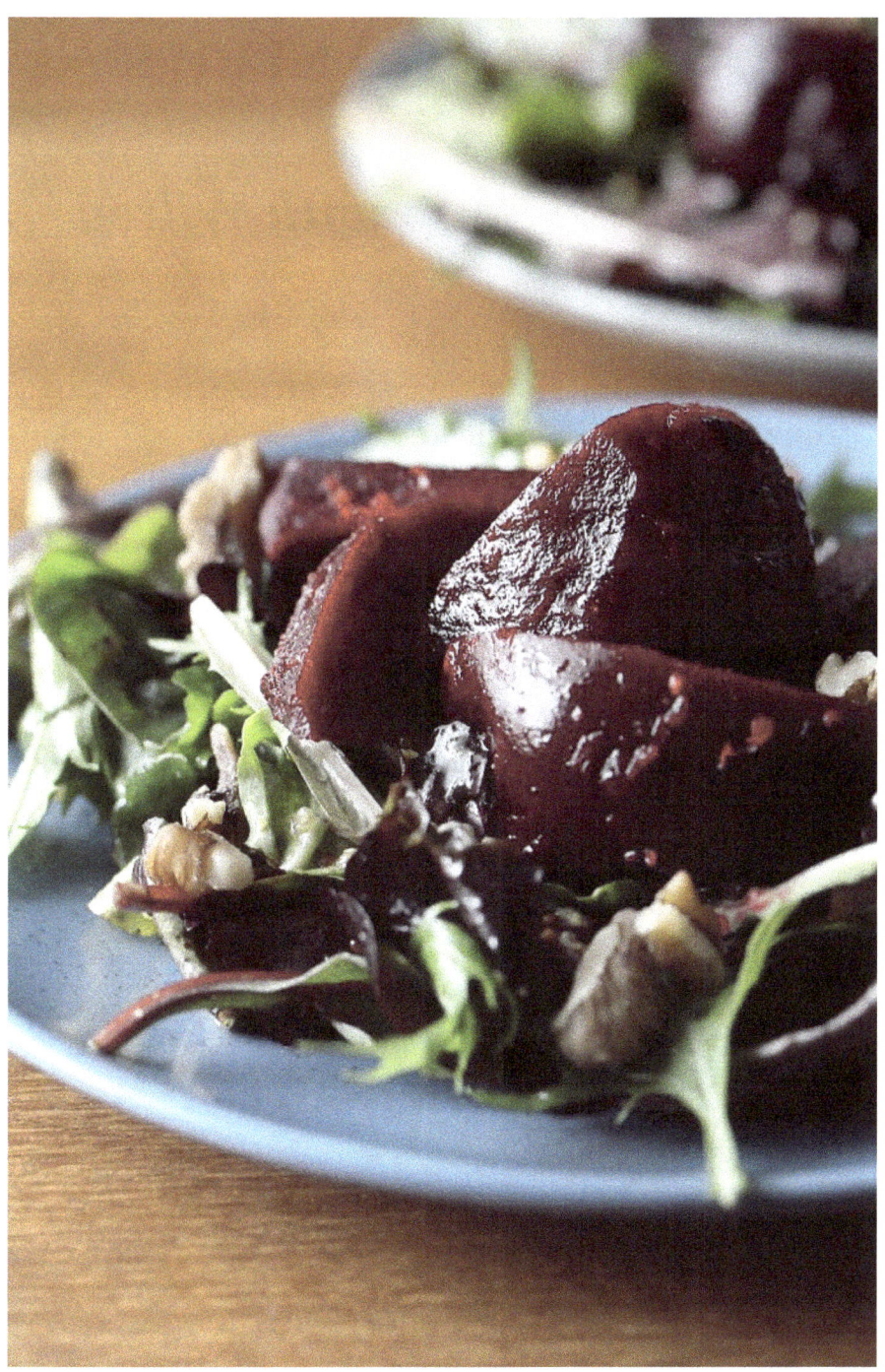

SOUPS AND STEWS

Quick Miso Soup with Wilted Greens

Time To Prepare: ten minutes
Time to Cook: five minutes
Yield: Servings 4

Ingredients:

- ½ teaspoon fish sauce
- 1 cup cut mushrooms
- 1 cup fresh baby spinach, meticulously washed
- 3 cups filtered water
- 3 cups vegetable broth
- 3 tablespoons miso paste
- 4 scallions, cut

Directions:

1. In a huge soup pot on high heat, put in the water, broth, mushrooms, and fish sauce, and bring to its boiling point. Turn off the heat.

2. In a small container, combine the miso paste with ½ cup of heated broth mixture to dissolve the miso. Mix the miso mixture back into the soup.
3. Mix in the spinach and scallions. Serve instantly.

Nutritional Info: Calories: 44 ‖ Total Fat: 0 ‖ Saturated Fat: 0g ‖ Cholesterol: 0mg ‖ Carbohydrates: 8g ‖ Fiber: 1g ‖ Protein: 2g

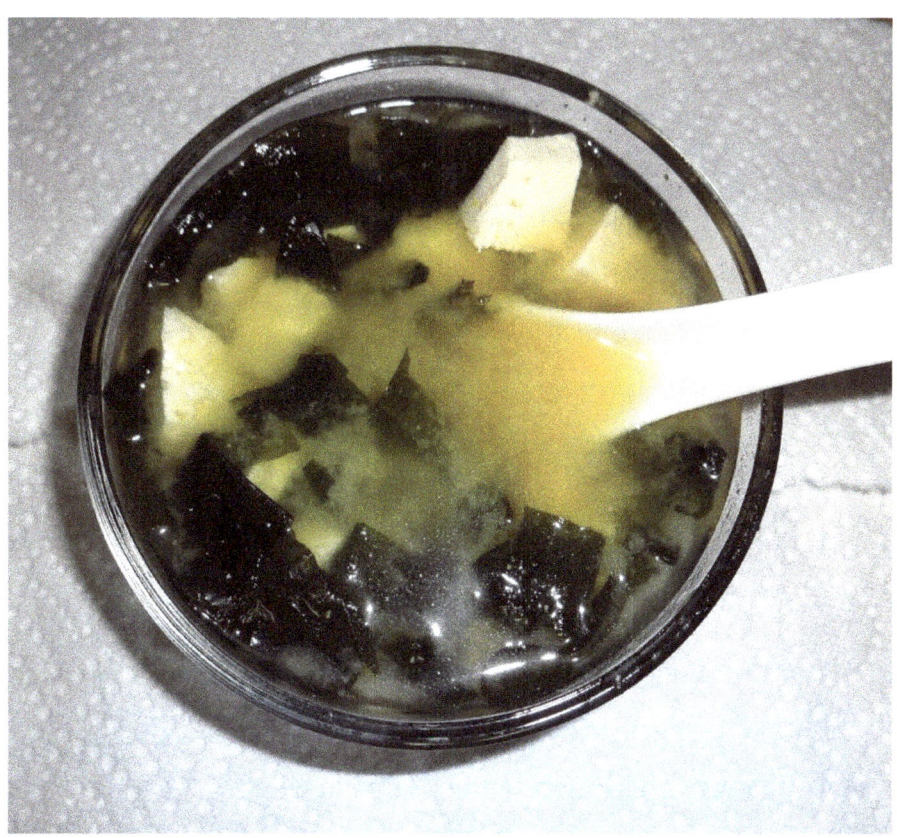

Red Lentil Dal

Time To Prepare: ten minutes
Time to Cook: twenty minutes
Yield: Servings 6

Ingredients:

- ½ teaspoon salt
- 1 (14-ounce) can unsweetened coconut milk
- 1 bay leaf
- 1 cup red dried lentils, sorted and washed well
- 1 medium tomato, diced
- 1 medium white onion, diced
- 1 tablespoon coconut oil
- 1 teaspoon ground cumin
- 1 teaspoon ground ginger
- 1 teaspoon ground turmeric
- 1 teaspoon mustard seeds
- 1 teaspoon sesame seeds
- 2 garlic cloves, minced
- 2 tablespoons chopped fresh cilantro leaves
- 3 cups vegetable broth
- Dash ground cinnamon

Directions:

1. In a huge soup pot using high heat, combine the broth, lentils, and bay leaf, and place to its boiling point. Lessen the heat to moderate-low and simmer for about twenty minutes, or until the lentils are cooked.
2. In the meantime, in a moderate-sized deep cooking pan on moderate heat, sauté the onion and garlic in the coconut oil for a couple of minutes.
3. Put in the tomato, sesame seeds, ginger, cumin, turmeric, mustard seeds, salt, and cinnamon. Cook, regularly stirring, for five minutes.
4. Mix in the coconut milk, then put it to a simmer.
5. Remove and discard the bay leaf. Put in the coconut milk mixture to the lentils together with the cilantro, and stir until blended. Serve alone or over rice if you wish.

Nutritional Info: Calories: 283 ∥ Total Fat: 6g ∥ Saturated Fat: 5g ∥ Cholesterol: 0mg ∥ Carbohydrates: 32g ∥ Fiber: 7g ∥ Protein: 14g

Ribollita

Time To Prepare: forty-five minutes
Time to Cook: 195 minutes
Yield: Servings 12

Ingredients:

- ½ Cup Olive Oil
- 1 Bunch Kale (Trimmed, Chopped)
- 1 Bunch Swiss Chard (Trimmed, Chopped)
- 1½ Cups Cabbage (Chopped)
- 12½ Inch-Thick Slices French Bread (Toasted)
- 2 Bay Leaves
- 2 Cups Dry Cannellini Beans (Rinsed)
- 2 Onions (Diced)
- 2 Potatoes (Peeled, Cut)
- 3 Carrots (Peeled, Sliced)
- 3 Large Stalks Celery (Chopped)
- 32 Ounce Chicken Broth
- 4 Cups Water
- 4 Sage Leaves
- 5 Cloves Garlic (Minced)
- Grated Parmesan Cheese
- Ground Black Pepper

- Ounce Tomatoes (Diced)
- Salt

Directions:

1. Boil beans in water for minimum five minutes and cool for 70 minutes.
2. Boil beans, garlic, sage leaves, bay leaves, and salt in chicken broth until soft.
3. Discard the leaves from half of the mixture.
4. Combine the remaining until the desired smoothness is achieved. Set aside.
5. Cook onions in oil, putting in carrots, potatoes, cabbage, celery, Swiss chard, and kale, tomatoes, and seasoning for about twenty minutes.
6. Put in the pureed bean and cook for forty minutes before you put in the rest of the mixture.
7. Put in toasted bread slices. Heat the soup for about twenty minutes.
8. Serve with Parmesan cheese and olive oil.

Nutritional Info: Calories: 418 kcal ‖ Carbohydrates: 41.8 g ‖ Fat: 22 g ‖ Protein: 14 g

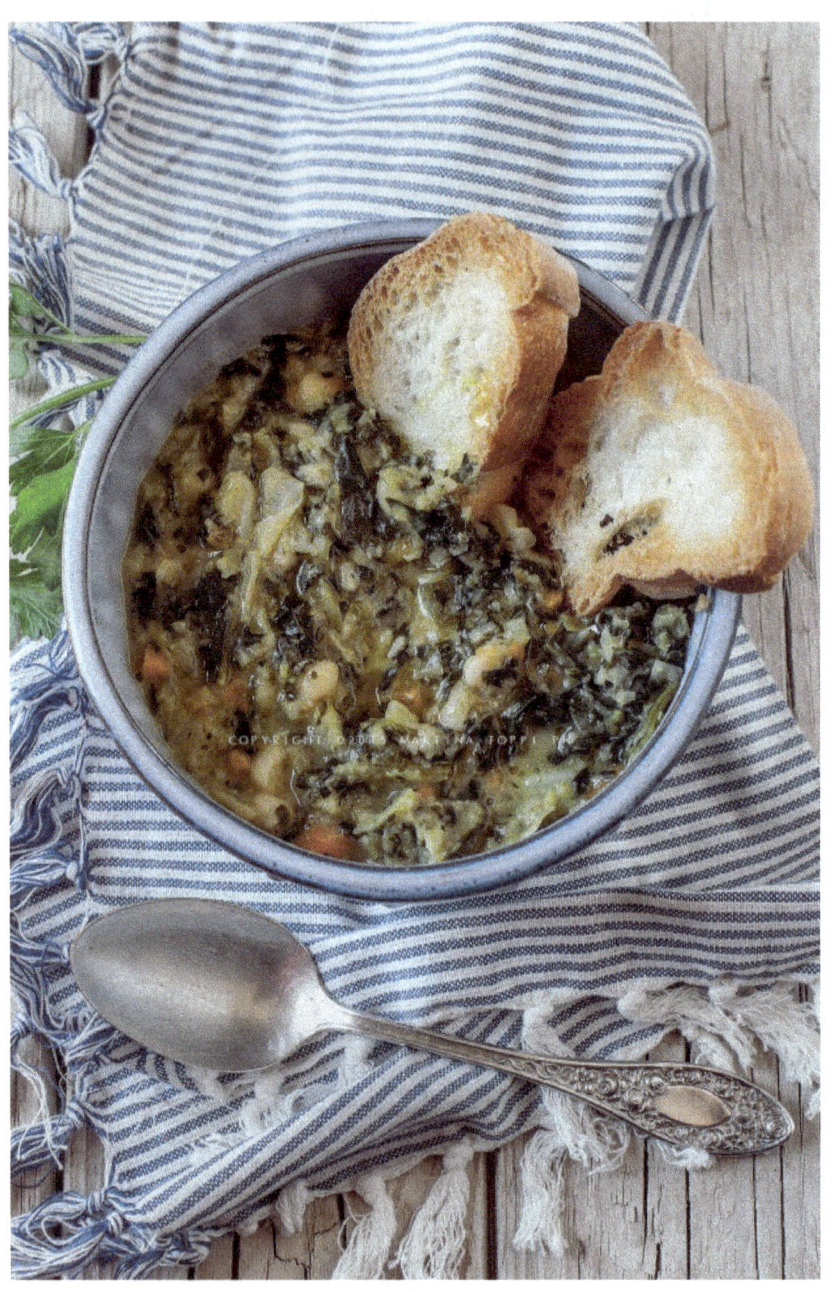

Rich Onion And Beef Stew

Time To Prepare: five minutes
Time to Cook: 10 hours
Yield: Servings 6

Ingredients:
- 1 beef stock cube
- 1 teaspoon dried mixed herbs (such as Italian seasoning)
- 2 onions, roughly chopped
- 2 pounds (907 g) boneless stewing beef, cut into cubes
- 3 cups water
- 3 tablespoons olive oil, divided
- 5 garlic cloves, crushed
- From the cupboard:
- Salt and freshly ground black pepper, to taste

Directions:
1. Grease the insert of the slow cooker with 2 tablespoons of olive oil. Coat a nonstick frying pan with the rest of the olive oil.
2. Heat the oil in the frying pan on moderate to high heat, then put the beef in the frying pan and sear for a couple

of minutes or until medium-rare. Shake the frying pan continuously to sear the beef cubes uniformly.
3. Position the cooked beef in the slow cooker, then put in the stock cube, mixed herbs, garlic, onions, salt, black pepper, and water. Stir to mix thoroughly.
4. Place the slow cooker lid on and cook on LOW for ten hours.
5. Ladle the stew in a big container and serve warm.

Nutritional Info: calories: 199 ∥ total fat: 6.3g ∥ carbs: 1.9g ∥ protein: 33.8g

Roasted Butternut Squash Apple Soup

Time To Prepare: ten minutes
Time to Cook: forty minutes
Yield: Servings 4

Ingredients:

- 1 butternut squash
- 1 celery rib
- 1 cup water
- 1 small onion
- 1/4 teaspoon cinnamon
- 1/4 teaspoon ginger
- 1/4 teaspoon nutmeg
- 2 red, sweet apples
- 3 cups low-sodium chicken/vegetable stock
- 4 tablespoons olive oil
- Salt & pepper to taste

Directions:

1. Preheat your oven to 400°F.
2. Put diced apple on a one-sheet pan & put the diced butternut squash on the second sheet pan.

3. Allow season to squash olive oil & put in pepper & salt. Stir get everything mix thoroughly. Put in apple with one tablespoon olive oil & stir to coat.
4. Apple & Roast squash for around half an hour, until browned.
5. Heat olive oil (remaining 1 ½ tablespoons) in a big stockpot.
6. Sauté celery & onion for around seven minutes, until soft. Put in Pepper & salt to taste.
7. Put in vegetable or chicken stock & water & bring to a simmer.
8. Once the apple & squash are roasted, put in them to the pot. Put in cinnamon, nutmeg & ginger.
9. Now blend the soup until the desired smoothness is achieved. Season pepper & salt to taste.
10. Serve with desired toppings.

Nutritional Info: Calories: 251 kcal ‖ Protein: 4.06 g ‖ Fat: 15.93 g ‖ Carbohydrates: 25.14 g

Russian Cabbage Soup (Shchi)

Time To Prepare: ten minutes
Time to Cook: twenty minutes
Yield: Servings 6

Ingredients:

- ½ big head cabbage, shredded
- ½ teaspoon salt
- 1 (14 oz.) can diced tomatoes with its juice
- 1 bay leaf
- 1 big potato, peeled and diced
- 1 celery stalk, diced
- 1 medium white onion, diced
- 1 tablespoon ghee
- 2 carrots, shredded
- 3 garlic cloves, minced
- 6 cups vegetable broth
- Freshly ground black pepper

Directions:

1. In a huge soup pot using high heat, mix the broth, bay leaf, and potato, and bring to its boiling point. Lower the heat to low and simmer for fifteen minutes.

2. In the meantime, in a moderate-sized deep cooking pan on moderate heat, heat the ghee. Place the onion and garlic, and sauté for five minutes.
3. Put in the carrots, celery, and cabbage, and cook for a couple of minutes, stirring frequently. Move to the soup pot.
4. Mix in the tomatoes and salt, and flavor with pepper. Mix thoroughly and carry on simmering until all ingredients have become tender and cooked, approximately five minutes. Take off and discard the bay leaf, and serve instantly.

Nutritional Info: Calories: 180 ∥ Total Fat: 3g ∥ Saturated Fat: 2g ∥ Cholesterol: 7mg ∥ Carbohydrates: 20g ∥ Fiber: 5g ∥ Protein: 12g

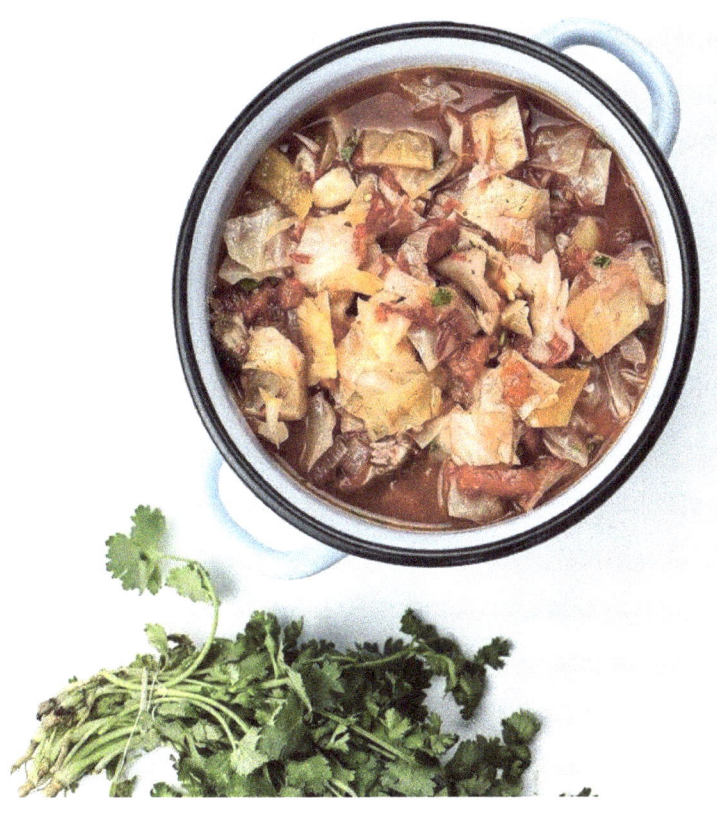

Saffron and Salmon Soup

Time To Prepare: ten minutes
Time to Cook: twenty minutes
Yield: Servings 4

Ingredients:

- ¼ cup extra-virgin olive oil
- ¼ tsp. freshly ground black pepper
- ¼ tsp. saffron threads
- ½ cup dry white wine
- 1 lb. salmon fillets, cut into 1-inch pieces
- 1 tsp. salt
- 2 cups baby spinach
- 2 garlic cloves, thinly cut
- 2 leeks, white parts only, thinly cut
- 2 medium carrots, thinly cut
- 2 tablespoons chopped scallions, both white and green parts
- 2 tablespoons finely chopped fresh flat-leaf parsley
- 4 cups vegetable broth

Directions:

1. In a large pot, heat the oil using high heat.

2. Put in the leeks, carrots, and garlic and sauté until tender, five to seven minutes.
3. Pour the broth then bring to its boiling point.
4. Reduce the heat to a simmer then put in the salmon, salt, pepper, and saffron. Cook until the salmon is thoroughly cooked, minimum 8 minutes.
5. Put in the spinach, wine, scallions, and parsley and cook until the spinach has wilted, one to two minutes, before you serve.

Nutritional Info: Calories: 418 ‖ Total Fat: 26g ‖ Total Carbohydrates: 13g ‖ Sugar: 4g ‖ Fiber: 2g ‖ Protein: 29g ‖ Sodium: 1455mg

Slow Cooker Lamb & Cauliflower Soup

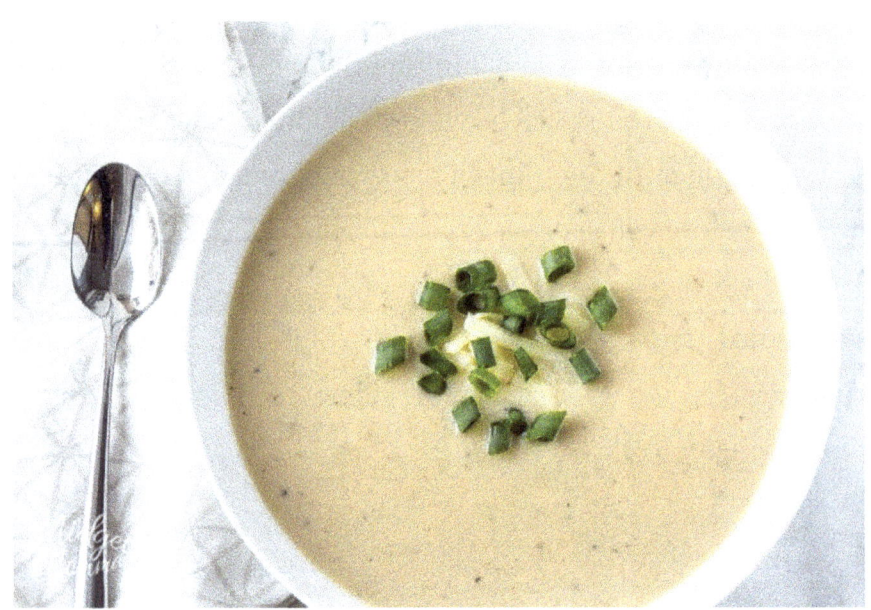

Time To Prepare: ten minutes
Time to Cook: 4 hours
Yield: Servings 6

Ingredients:

- ½ teaspoon cracked black pepper
- ½ teaspoon salt
- 1 cauliflower head, cut into florets

- 1 cup heavy cream
- 1 pound ground lamb
- 1 tablespoon freshly chopped thyme
- 1 yellow onion, chopped
- 2 cloves garlic, chopped
- 5 cups beef broth

Directions:
1. Put in the ground lamb and cauliflower to the base of a stockpot.
2. Put in in the rest of the ingredients minus the heavy cream, and cook on high for 4 hours.
3. Warm the heavy cream before you put in to the soup. Use an immersion blender to combine the soup until creamy.

Nutritional Info: Calories: 263 ‖ Carbohydrates: 6g ‖ Fiber: 2g Net ‖ Carbohydrates: 4g ‖ Fat: 14g ‖ Protein: 27g

Spicy Asian-Style Soup

Time To Prepare: ten minutes
Yield: Servings 4

Ingredients:

- ½ cup soy milk
- ½ pound asparagus, diced
- 1 bay leaf
- 1 cup celery, diced
- 1 shallot, diced
- 1 tablespoon coconut aminos
- 1 teaspoon Taco seasoning
- 1/4 teaspoon freshly ground black pepper
- 2 chicken bouillon cubes
- 2 cloves garlic, diced
- 2 cups Crimini mushrooms
- 2 tablespoons butter, softened
- 4 cups water
- Sea salt and black pepper, to taste

Directions:

1. Push the "Sauté" button to heat up your Instant Pot. Once hot, melt the butter; then, sweat the shallot until tender.

2. Mix in garlic; cook an additional 40 seconds, stirring regularly.
3. Put in the rest of the ingredients.
4. Secure the lid. Choose "Manual" mode and High pressure; cook for seven minutes. Once cooking is complete, use a quick pressure release; cautiously remove the lid.
5. Ladle into separate bowls and serve warm. Enjoy!

Nutritional Info: 104 Calories ‖ 7g Fat ‖ 6.6g Total Carbs ‖ 3.9g Protein ‖ 3.5g Sugars

DESSERTS

Pumpkin Ice Cream

Time To Prepare: fifteen minutes
Time to Cook: 0 minutes
Yield: Servings 6

Ingredients:

- ½ cup of dates (pitted and chopped)
- ½ teaspoon of ground cinnamon
- ½ teaspoon of vanilla flavor
- 1 (fifteen-ounce) can of sugar-free pumpkin puree
- 1 ½ teaspoon of pumpkin pie spice
- 2 (14-ounce) cans of unsweetened coconut milk
- Pinch of salt

Directions:

1. Combine all ingredients in a high-speed blender and pulse.
2. Move the puree to an airtight container and freeze for roughly 1-2 hours.
3. Move the frozen puree to an ice-cream maker and process following the manufacturers.

4. Return the ice-cream to the airtight container and freeze for approximately 1-2 hours before you serve.

Nutritional Info: ‖ Calories: 373 ‖ Fat: 31.9g ‖ Carbohydrates: 24.7g ‖ Sugar: 16.2g ‖ Protein: 4.2g ‖ Sodium: 51mg

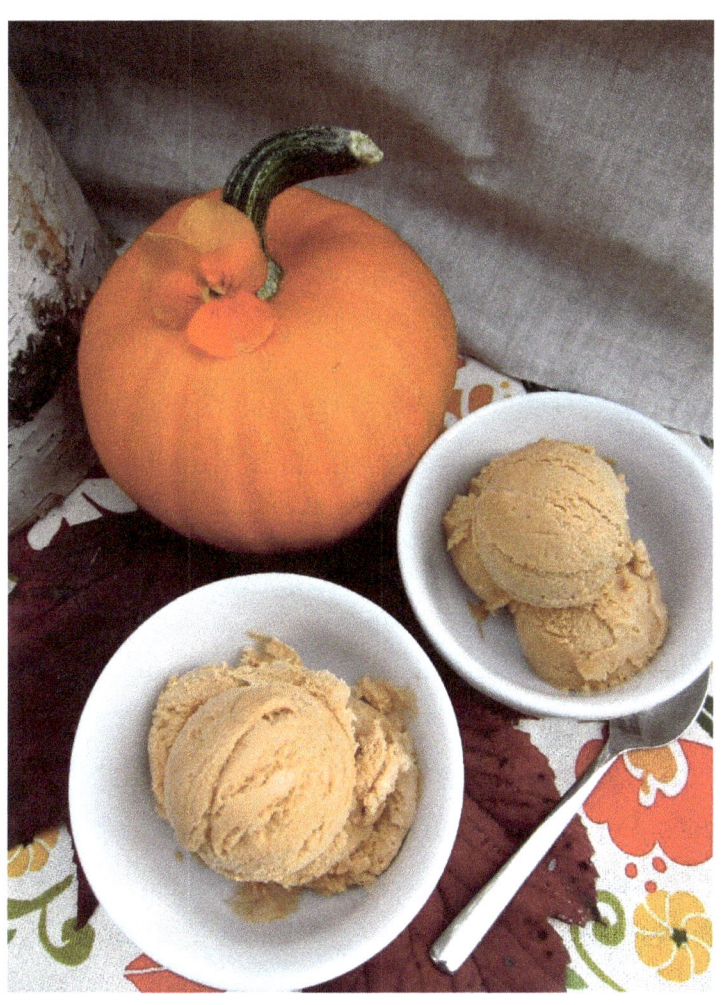

Pure Avocado Pudding

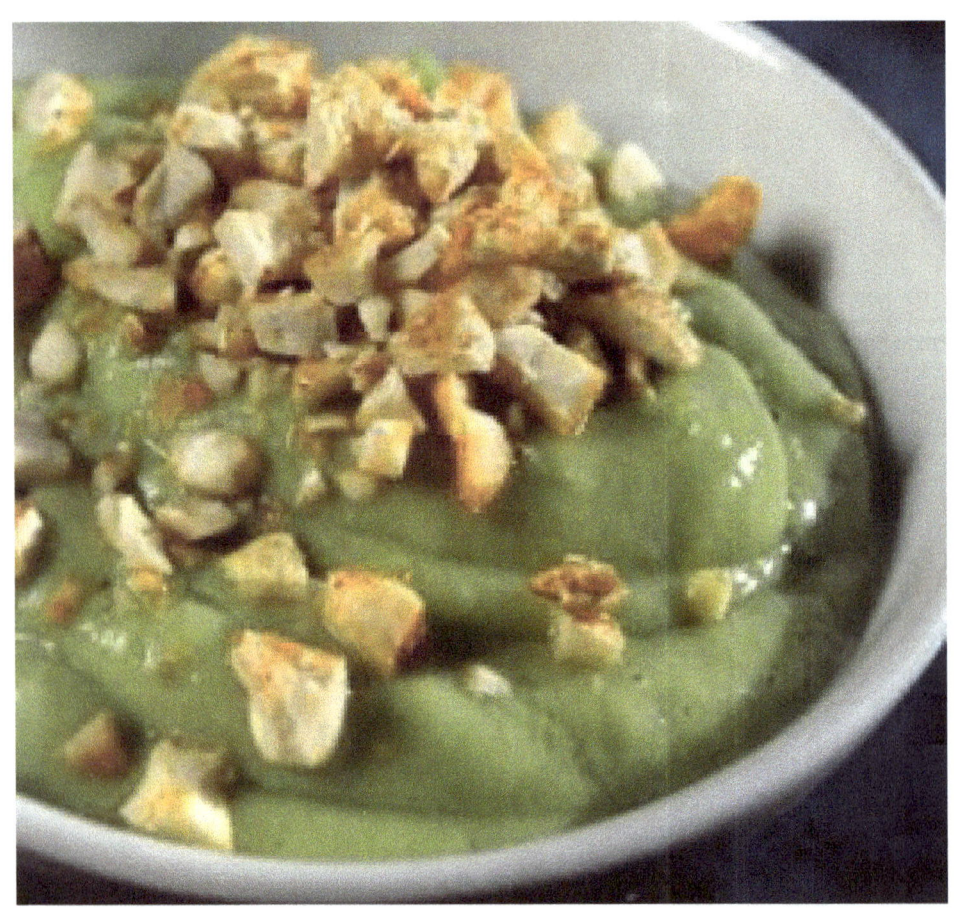

Time To Prepare: three hours
Time to Cook: 0 minutes
Yield: Servings 4

Ingredients:

- ¼ teaspoon cinnamon
- ¾ cup cocoa powder
- 1 cup almond milk
- 1 teaspoon vanilla extract
- 2 avocados, peeled and pitted
- 2 tablespoons stevia
- Walnuts, chopped for serving

Directions:

1. Put in avocados to a blender and pulse well
2. Put in cocoa powder, almond milk, stevia, vanilla bean extract and pulse the mixture well
3. Put into serving bowls then top with walnuts
4. Chill for two to three hours and serve!

Nutritional Info: ‖ Calories: 221 ‖ Fat: 8g ‖ Carbohydrates: 7g ‖ Protein: 3g

Raspberry Diluted Frozen Sorbet

Time To Prepare: 10 min
Time to Cook: 20 min
Yield: Servings 4

Ingredients:

- 1 tsp honey
- 14oz / 400g frozen raspberry
- fl oz / 50g almond milk
- Mint

Directions:

1. Place the almond milk and raspberry in a mixer till it's smooth and leave the consistency in the freezer for about twenty minutes.
2. When serving, place them in ice cream bowls and serve with mint on top.

Nutritional Info: ‖ Calories: 47 ‖ Carbohydrates: 11 g ‖ Protein: 1 g ‖ Fat: 0.4 g ‖ Sugar: 37.2 g ‖ Fiber: 6.0 g ‖ Sodium: 24 mg

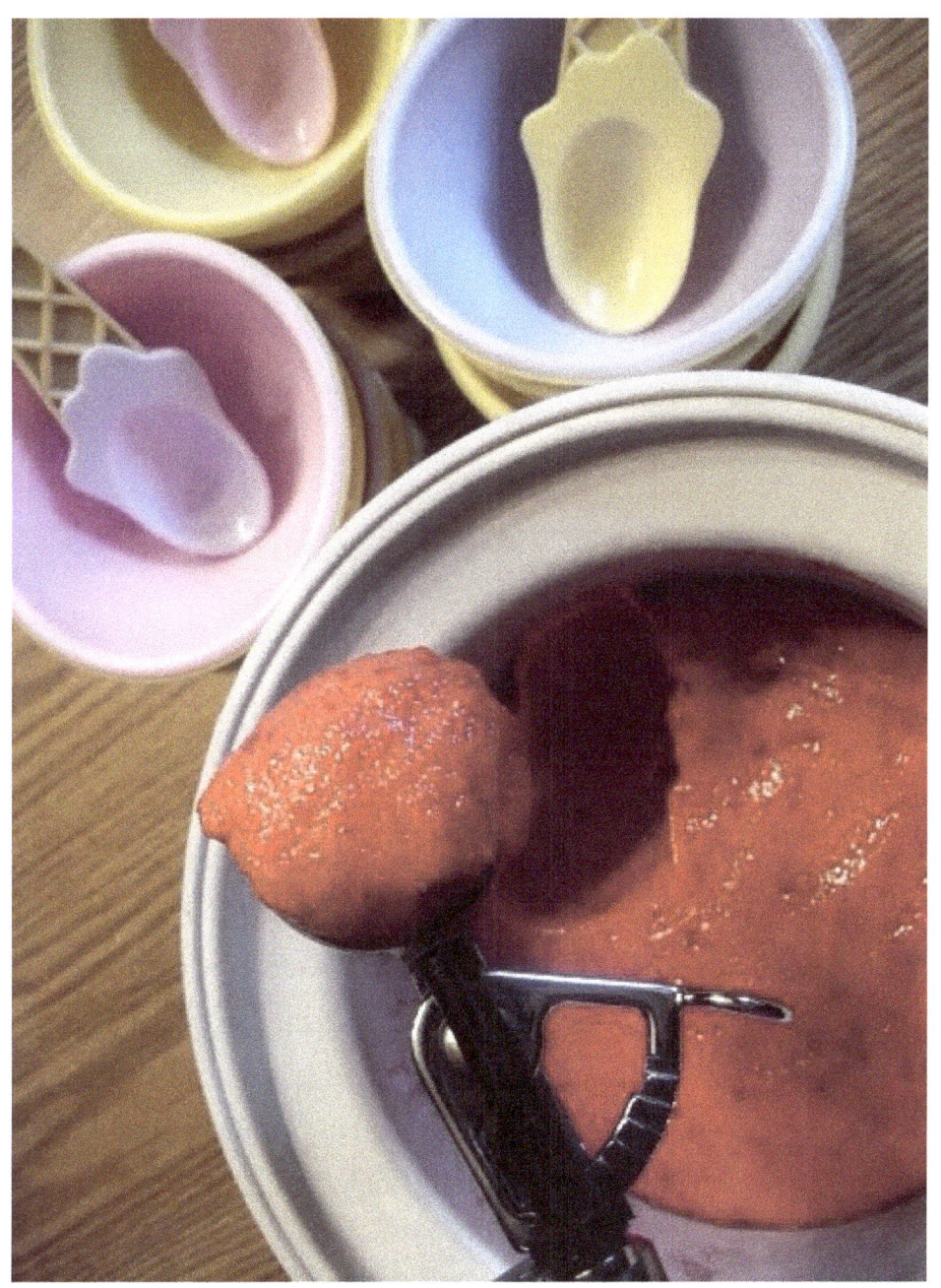

Raspberry Gummies

Time To Prepare: five minutes
Time to Cook: fifteen minutes
Yield: Servings 6

Ingredients:

- ¼ cup of grass-fed gelatin
- ¾ cup of cold water
- 1 cup of frozen raspberries
- 3 tablespoons of raw honey

Directions:

1. Put the water and frozen raspberries into a blender, and blend until the desired smoothness is achieved. Put into a big deep cooking pan on moderate heat.
2. Put in the honey and gelatin and whisk together. Reduce the heat, then whisk for another five minutes.
3. Pour into molds or a baking dish, and place in your fridge for minimum 1 hour until firm. If you use a baking dish, chop the gelatin into squares; if not, just pop the gelatin out of the molds.

Nutritional Info: ‖ Total Carbohydrates: 9g ‖ Fiber: 1g ‖ Net Carbohydrates: ‖ Protein: 0g ‖ Total Fat: 0g ‖ Calories: 37

Raspberry Gummies

Time To Prepare: five minutes
Time to Cook: fifteen minutes
Yield: Servings 6

Ingredients:

- ¼ cup of grass-fed gelatin
- ¾ cup of cold water
- 1 cup of frozen raspberries
- 3 tablespoons of raw honey

Directions:

1. Pour water into a blender followed by frozen raspberries. Puree and move them to a deep cooking pan on moderate heat.
2. Put in honey and gelatin. Whisk. Reduce the heat, then whisk constantly for five minutes.
3. Place the mixture on a baking dish or molds and place in your fridge for 60 minutes or until it firms.
4. If you used a baking dish, chop the gelatin into squares. Pop the gelatin out with the molds.

Nutritional Info: ‖ Total Carbohydrates: 9g ‖ Fiber: 1g ‖ Protein: 0g ‖ Total Fat: 0g ‖ Calories: 37

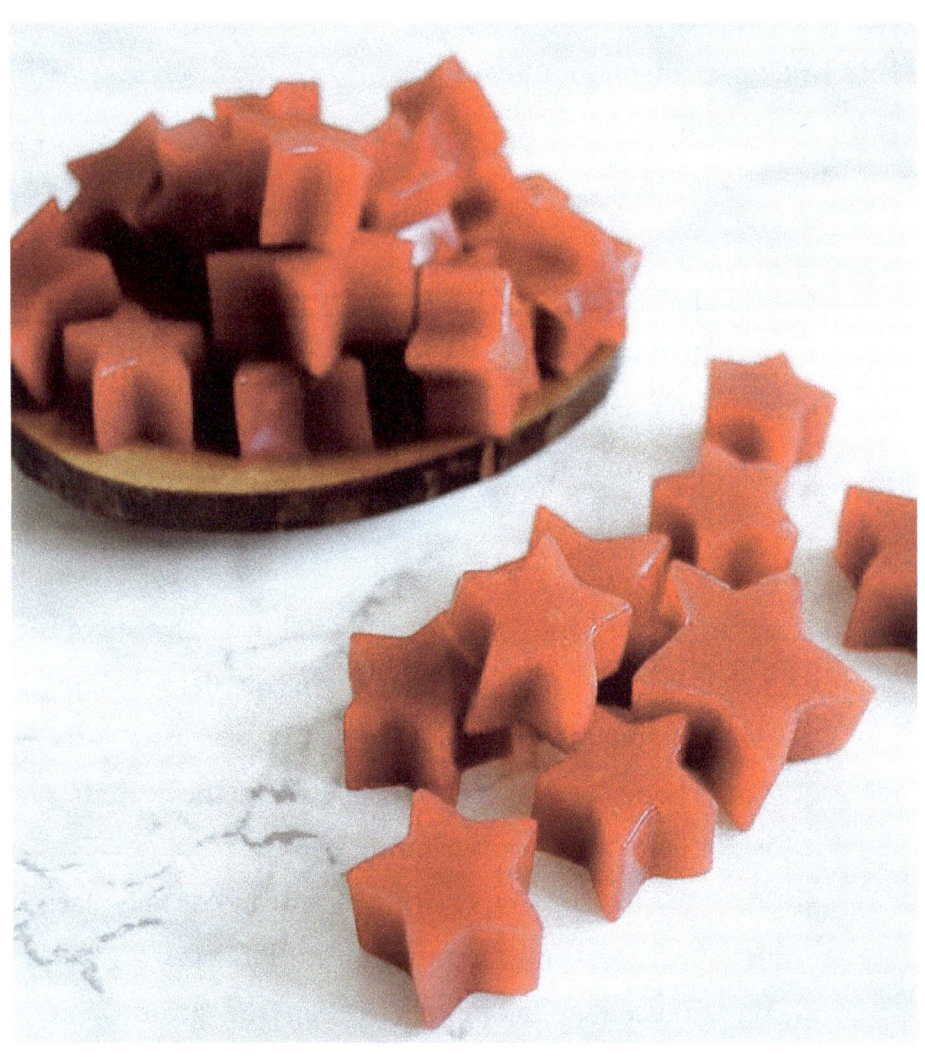

Raw Black Forest Brownies

Time To Prepare: 2 hours and ten minutes
Time to Cook: 0 minute
Yield: Servings 6

Ingredients:
- ¼ teaspoon salt
- ½ cup almonds, chopped
- ½ cup dates pitted
- 1 and ½ cups cherries, pitted, dried and chopped
- 1 cup raw cacao powder
- 2 cups walnuts, chopped

Directions:
1. Put all ingredients in a food processor
2. Pulse until small crumbs are formed
3. Push the brownie batter in a pan
4. Freeze for a couple of hours
5. Slice before you serve and enjoy!

Nutritional Info: ‖ Calories: 294 ‖ Fat: 18g ‖ Carbohydrates: 33g ‖ Protein: 7g

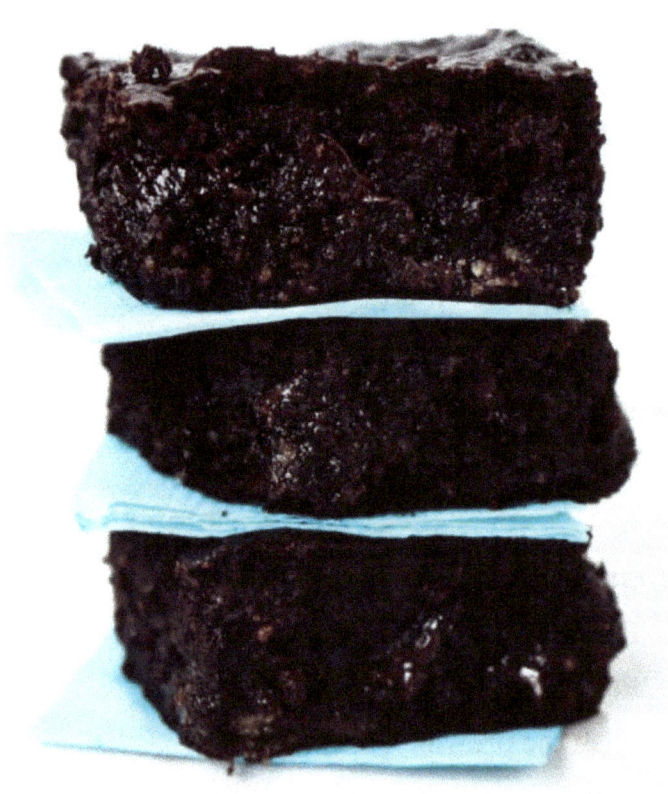

Refreshing Raspberry Jelly

Time To Prepare: ten minutes+ 1 hour freezing
Time to Cook: thirty minutes
Yield: Servings 4

Ingredients:

- ¼ cup of water
- 1 tbsp. of fresh lemon juice
- 2 pound of fresh raspberries

Directions:

1. In a moderate-sized pan, put in raspberries and water on low heat and cook for approximately 8-ten minutes until done completely.
2. Put in lemon juice and cook for approximately 30 minutes, stirring once in a while.
3. Turn off the heat and put the mixture into a sieve.
4. Position a strainer over a container.
5. Through strainer, strain the mixture by pushing using the backside of a spoon.
6. Place the mixture into a blender then pulse till a jelly-like texture is formed.
7. Move into serving glass bowls and place in your fridge for minimum for approximately 1 hour.

Nutritional Info: ‖ Calories: 119 ‖ Fat: 1.5g ‖ Carbohydrates: 27.2g ‖ Protein: 2.8g ‖ Fiber: 14.8g

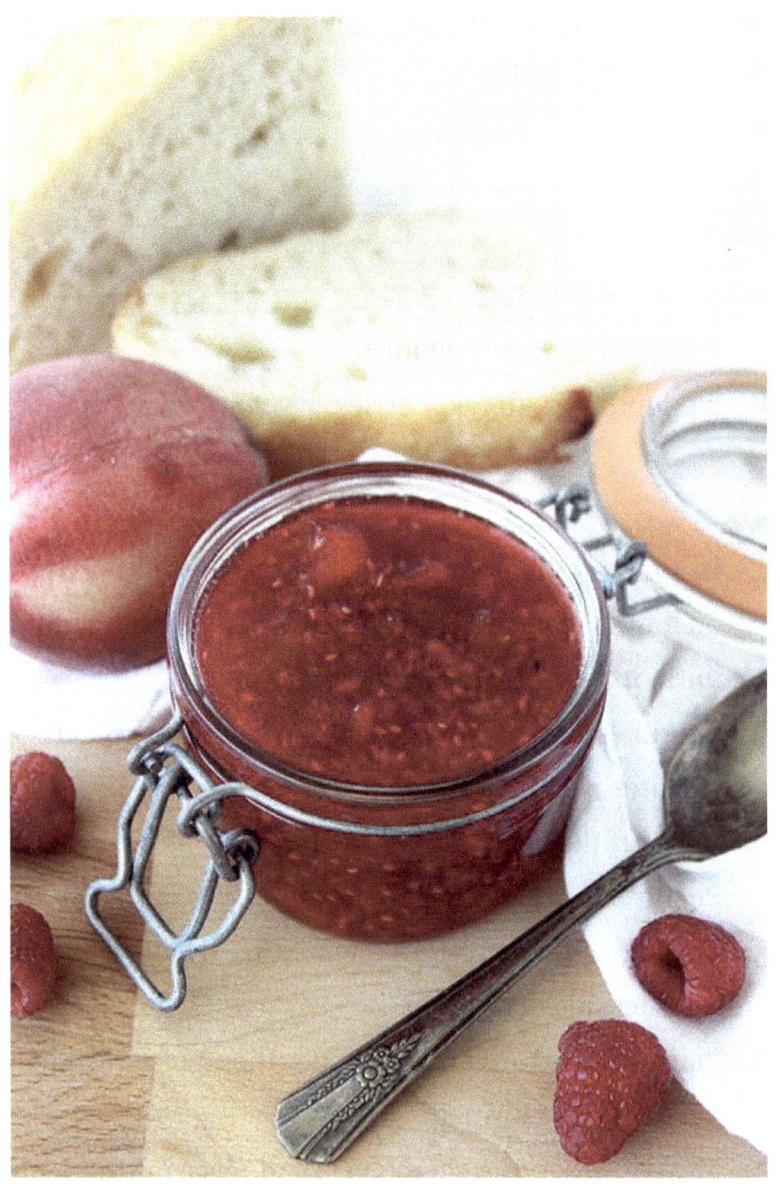

Roasted Bananas

Time To Prepare: two minutes
Time to Cook: seven minutes
Yield: Servings 1

Ingredients:

- 1 banana, cut into diagonal pieces
- Avocado oil cooking spray

Directions:

1. Take parchment paper and line the air fryer basket with it.
2. Preheat the air fryer to 190 degrees C or 375 degrees F.
3. Keep your slices of banana in the basket. Make sure they do not touch
4. Apply avocado oil to mist the slices of banana.
5. Cook for five minutes.
6. Take out the basket. Flip the slices cautiously.
7. Cook for two more minutes. The slices of banana must be caramelized and brown. Remove them from the basket.

Nutritional Info: Calories 121 ‖ Carbohydrates: 27g ‖ Cholesterol: 0mg ‖ Total Fat: 1g ‖ Protein: 1g ‖ Sugar: 14g ‖ Fiber: 3g ‖ Sodium: 1mg

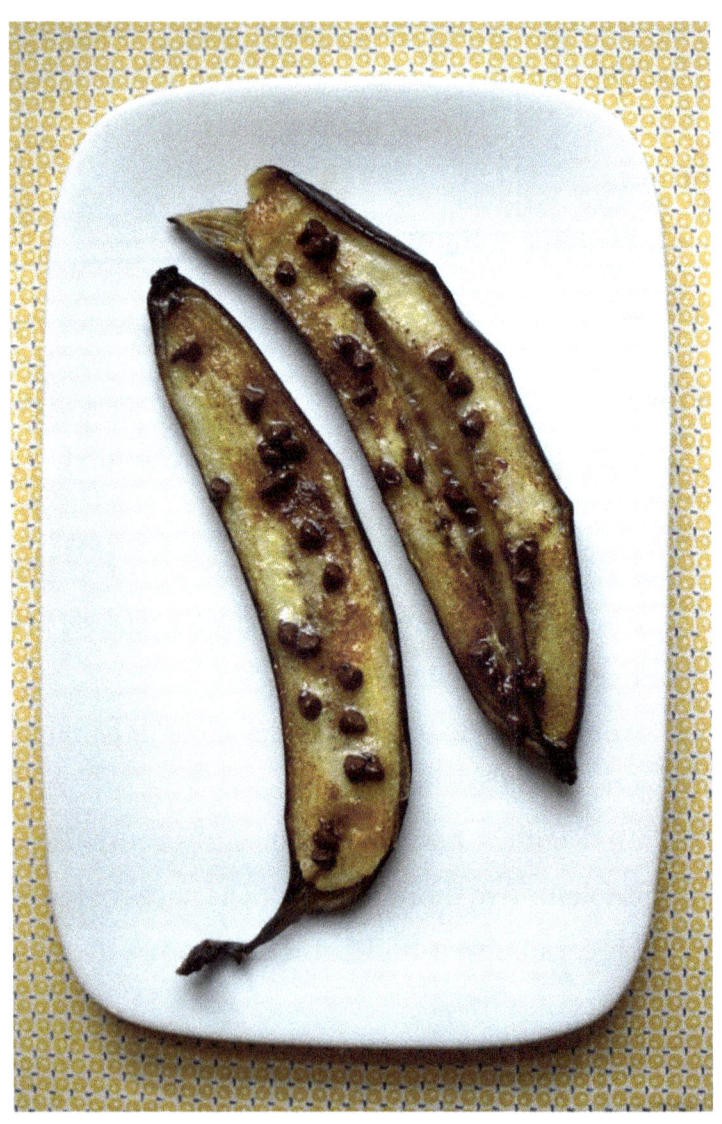

Rum Butter Cookies

Time To Prepare: ten minutes + chilling time
Time to Cook: five minutes
Yield: Servings 12

Ingredients:

- ½ cup coconut butter
- ½ cup confectioners' Swerve
- 1 stick butter
- 1 teaspoon rum extract
- 4 cups almond meal

Directions:

1. Melt the coconut butter and butter. Mix in the Swerve and rum extract.
2. Afterward, put in in the almond meal and mix to blend.
3. Roll the balls and put them on a parchment-lined cookie sheet.
4. Keep in your fridge until ready to serve.

Nutritional Info: 400 Calories 40g ‖ Fat: 4.9g ‖ Carbs: 5.4g ‖ Protein: 2.9g

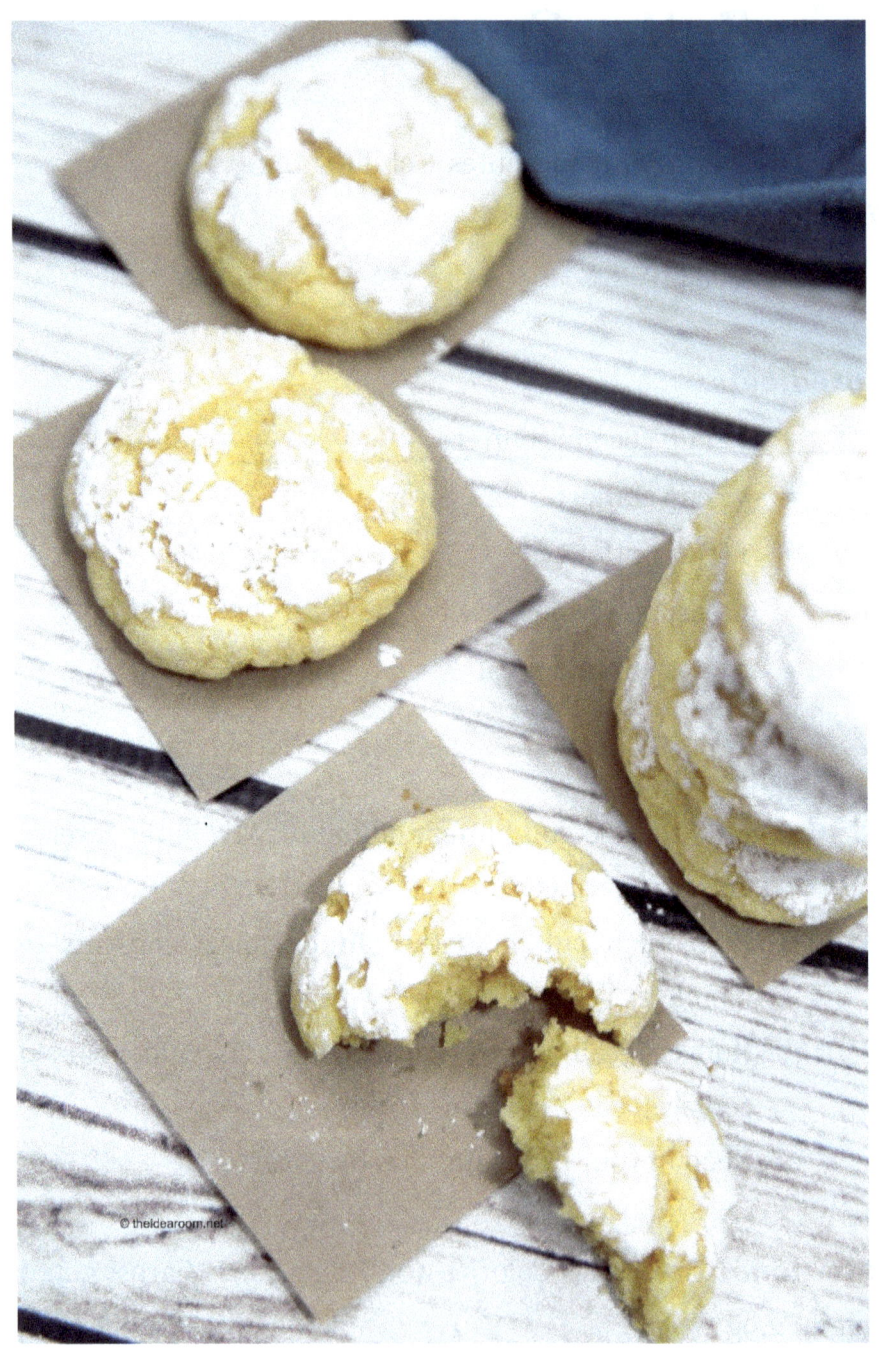

Sherbet Pineapple

Time To Prepare: 20 Minutes
Time to Cook: 0 Minute
Yield: Servings 4

Ingredients:

- 1 can of 8-ounce pineapple chunks
- ¼ teaspoon of ground ginger
- ¼ teaspoon of vanilla extract
- 1 can of 11-ounce orange sections
- 2 cups of pineapple, lemon or lime sherbet
- 1/3 cup of orange marmalade

Directions:

1. Drain the pineapple, ensure you reserve the juice.
2. Take a moderate-sized container and put in pineapple juice, ginger, vanilla and marmalade to the container
3. Put in pineapple chunks, drained mandarin oranges as well
4. Toss thoroughly and coat everything
5. Free them for fifteen minutes and let them chill
6. Ladle the sherbet into 4 chilled stemmed sherbet dishes
7. Top each of them with fruit mixture

Enjoy!

Nutritional Info: ‖ Calories: 267 Cal ‖ Fat: 1 g ‖ Carbohydrates: 65 g ‖ Protein: 2 g

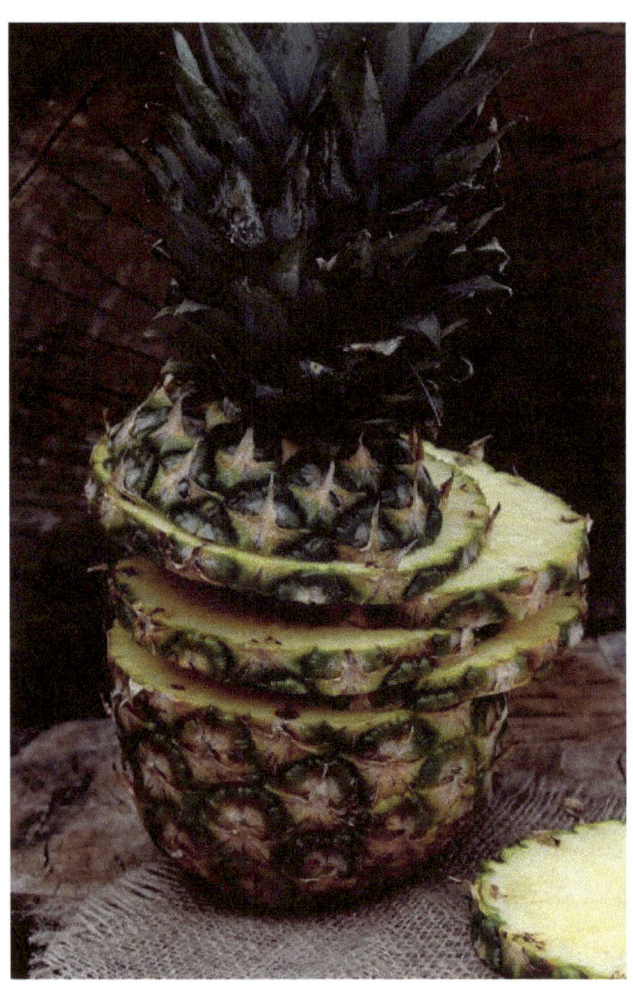

www.ingramcontent.com/pod-product-compliance
Lightning Source LLC
Chambersburg PA
CBHW071107030426
42336CB00013BA/1988